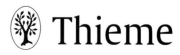

Practical
MR Mammography

Uwe Fischer, M.D.

Women's Health Care Center
Goettingen, Germany

With the collaboration of Ulrich Brinck, M.D.

398 illustrations
25 tables

Thieme
Stuttgart · New York

Library of Congress Cataloging-in-Publication Data

This book is an authorized translation of the German edition published and copyrighted 2000 by Georg Thieme Verlag, Stuttgart, Germany. Title of the German edition: Lehratlas der MR-Mammographie

Collaborator:
Ulrich Brinck, M.D.
Department of Pathology
University Hospital
Göttingen, Germany

Translator: Dr. Susanne Luftner Nagel, Göttingen, Germany

Important note: Medicine is an ever-changing science undergoing continual development. Research and clinical experience are continually expanding our knowledge, in particular our knowledge of proper treatment and drug therapy. Insofar as this book mentions any dosage or application, readers may rest assured that the authors, editors, and publishers have made every effort to ensure that such references are in accordance with **the state of knowledge at the time of production of the book.**
Nevertheless, this does not involve, imply, or express any guarantee or responsibility on the part of the publishers in respect to any dosage instructions and forms of applications stated in the book. **Every user is requested to examine carefully** the manufacturers' leaflets accompanying each drug and to check, if necessary in consultation with a physician or specialist, whether the dosage schedules mentioned therein or the contraindications stated by the manufacturers differ from the statements made in the present book. Such examination is particularly important with drugs that are either rarely used or have been newly released on the market. Every dosage schedule or every form of application used is entirely at the user's own risk and responsibility. The authors and publishers request every user to report to the publishers any discrepancies or inaccuracies noticed.

© 2004 Georg Thieme Verlag,
Rüdigerstrasse 14, 70469 Stuttgart, Germany
http://www.thieme.de
Thieme New York, 333 Seventh Avenue,
New York, NY 10001 USA
http://www.thieme.com

Typesetting by primustpe R. Hurler GmbH,
D-73274 Notzingen

Printed in Germany by Staudigl-Druck,
D-86609 Donauwörth

ISBN 3-13-132031-1 (GTV)
ISBN 1-58890-168-8 (TNY)   1 2 3 4 5

Foreword

Mammography has a long-standing tradition in Göttingen. Anton Gregl founded and established conventional diagnostic radiography of the breast at the university clinic here in the 1970s. He based his work on the „Strassburg school of senology" and upon the experience of Becker in Heidelberg, as well as that of Hoeffken and Lanyi in Cologne. As a consequence of his great merits, an independent department for mammography and lymphology was conferred on him. He remained head of this department. until his retirement in 1989.

It was in this department that Uwe Fischer began his education in radiology. After Professor Gregl's retirement and the reintegration of this specialized department into the department of diagnostic radiology, it seemed reasonable to increase the use of modern sectional imaging methods for the detection of breast cancer. Besides the performance of ultrasonography, special interest was given to the use of MR mammography following the fundamental research been done by Heywang and Kaiser since 1986.

After the first MR unit was put into operation at our clinic in the 1990's, Uwe Fischer took advantage of his experience in conventional mammography from the Gregl era, and of this opportunity to validate the clinical value of MR mammography on a large patient population. This textbook is the result of his nine years of experience and endeavor in this field. It covers the generally accepted spectrum of indications, recommendations in the area of technique and methods, and current knowledge of the morphological and hemodynamic findings, as well as possibilities for relevant interventional diagnostics and therapy. During the years of Uwe Fischer's clinical and scientific activities, which also led to his habilitation, he has substantially contributed to furthering the acknowledgment of our clinic and strengthening its reputation. Uwe Fischer is thus especially qualified to write an up-to-date, critical compendium of MR mammography. It is with great happiness that I see this book finished and I hope it will be a helpful and widely enjoyed addition to the libraries of our interested colleagues.

Göttingen   Prof. Dr. Eckhardt Grabbe

Preface

In recent years, dynamic MR mammography has increasingly established itself as an imaging modality in the diagnostic work-up of the female breast. As a complementary method, it fills an important gap that remains despite numerous technical improvements and developments in the areas of x-ray mammography and ultrasonography of the breast. The approach particular to contrast-enhanced MR mammography allows the visualization of pathological tissue hypervascularization, which permits the detection of invasive breast cancer with high sensitivity.

In spite of the great initial controversies surrounding the methodology of MR examinations, general agreement on a standardized examination strategy has been achieved in the European community in recent years. The current guidelines, published in the form of recommendations by the Deutsche Röntgengesellschaft (DRG)—the German radiological society—represent a consensus of many work groups. The fact that the measurement protocols of individual researchers still show certain differences in some parameters does not contradict this. Instead, this should be considered a demonstration of the manifold possibilities that magnetic resonance imaging (MRI) has to offer.

MRI of the breast is an additional method available to radiologists that, if performed selectively, can improve the diagnostic imaging of breast cancer. If heed is taken of a defined catalogue of indications, the cost-avalanche feared by some can be avoided. On the contrary, one can expect that its selective use will allow tumors and recurrences to be recognized earlier, and the subsequent planning and performance of therapeutic procedures to be better adapted to the tumor stage.

It is the goal of this book to be an introduction to and a compendium of MR mammography, as well as an aid in the daily routine dealings with the method. The important technical and methodological aspects of MR mammography are presented in short and concise form. One chapter is devoted exclusively to the evaluation criteria. This treatment is completed by a description of the physiological changes of the breast and a discussion of potential artifacts and pitfalls.

The main emphasis of the book is on providing a systematic account of changes and diseases relevant to breast diagnostics. As an introduction, the most important information regarding histology, epidemiology, prognosis, and clinical significance of breast diseases, as well as imaging with other modalities, is presented. This short outline does not represent a complex discourse on the specific findings, but should serve as a quick review.

For more detailed information, it will be necessary to refer to relevant literature on the subject. The following chapter is dedicated to specifying generally accepted indications for the performance of contrast-enhanced MR mammography. Examples are illustrated with impressive images.

A separate chapter is devoted to the analysis of MRI findings in combination with the findings of other breast imaging modalities. Recommendations pertaining to diagnostic and therapeutic strategies in MR mammography are intended to give practical guidance for daily routine practice and are not meant to be a rigid book of rules to which one must adhere. The more experienced reader may be dissatisfied in particular with some parts of this chapter because of its brevity. However, it is the pragmatic approach of this chapter, which does not take into consideration the least frequently encountered differential diagnoses, that will make it of valuable assistance in reaching the correct diagnosis.

The basics of performing MR mammography on patients with breast implants, and the imaging of typical complications are described together in one chapter. A discussion of the current stand on MR-guided interventional techniques, which can occasionally be required for the prompt clarification of findings, and comments on quality assurance as well as perspectives for the future complete and conclude the subject of MR mammography.

This book reflects the twelve years of experience in MR mammography that I have acquired in the department of diagnostic radiology at the Georg-August University Göttingen. Such a project is inconceivable without the contributions of many fellow-workers. At this point I would therefore like to thank Ms. Margitta Pieper, whose untiring patience provided for the high-quality photographic reproductions. I thank all the medical technologists in the department, with special mention of Ms. Jutta Rüschoff and Mr. Thomas Weidlich, who attended to the many patients during their MR examination with remarkable consideration and enthusiasm. More thanks go to Dr. Corinna Schorn, who worked on special aspects of MR mammography with innovative ideas and meticulous care, and to Dr. Dorit von Heyden and Dr. Susanne Luftner-Nagel, who performed most of the clinical, mammographic, and ultrasonographic examinations before MR mammography. I am especially grateful to Prof. Dr. Alfred Schauer of the pathology department of the Georg-August University Göttingen, who was always available for constructive discussions, and PD Dr. Ulrich Brinck of the same pathology department, who wrote the sections on histopathology and immunhistochemistry and contributed the respective histological slides. My heart-felt thanks go to Dr. Werner Döler of the medical physics department for the good cooperation in planning and building MRI compatible equipment. Finally, my special thanks go to two people: first, to my teacher and mentor Prof. Dr. Anton Gregl, who introduced me to breast diagnostics 19 years ago with contagious enthusiasm and passion; second, to Prof. Dr. Eckhardt Grabbe, who made it possible for me to concentrate on clinical and scientific research involving MRI of the breast, and always supported my endeavors constructively.

Göttingen, summer of 2003   Uwe Fischer

Contents

Abbreviations

ACR	American College of Radiology	LCIS	Lobular carcinoma in situ
bFGF	Basic fibroblast growth factor	LE	Lumpectomy
BW	Body weight	LN	Lymph node
cc	Cranio-caudal	ml	Medio-lateral
CD	Cluster determinants	ms	Millisecond
CE	Contrast-enhanced	MIP	Maximum intensity projection
CM	Contrast material	MPR	Multiplanar reconstruction
2D	Data acquisition in single slices	MR	Magnetic resonance
3D	Data acquisition in volume block	MRI	Magnetic resonance imaging
DCIS	Ductal carcinoma in situ	NMR	Nuclear magnetic resonance
DD	Differential diagnosis	NOS	Not otherwise specified
DRG	Deutsche Röntgengesellschaft	NU	Normalized units
DTPA	Diethylenetriamine pentaacetic acic; pentetic acid	OP	Operation
		PEG	Phase encoded gradient
EIC	Extensive intraductal component	Post-CM	After contrast administration
FA	Flip angle	Pre-CM	Before contrast administration
FLASH	Fast low-angle shot	RODEO	Rotating Delivery of Excitation Off Resonance
FOV	Field of view		
G	Gauge	ROI	Region of interest
G 1,2,3	Grade 1,2,3	SE	Sample excision
Gd	Gadolinium	SE	Spin echo
Gd-DTPA	Gadolinium-DTPA	T	Tesla (unit of magnetic field strength)
GE	Gradient echo	T1-WI	T1-weighted
Gy	Gray (unit of absorbed dose/energy of radiation)	T2-WI	T2-weighted
		TE	Time-to-echo
HPF	High-power field	TNM	Tumor–node–metastasis staging system
HR	High-resolution	TR	Time-to-repetition
IIBM	International investigation of breast MR imaging (international multicenter study)	TSE	Turbo-spin-echo
		TurboFLASH	Ultrafast GE sequence
IR	Inversion recovery	VEGF	Vascular endothelial growth factor

1 History of MR Mammography

The development of magnetic resonance imaging (MRI) was set off by the work of the chemist Paul Lauterbur in the early 1970s. On the basis of the research of Bloch and Purcell, it was Lauterbur who made possible spatial encoding within a static magnetic field by using linear variations of field strength along the spatial coordinates (Lauterbur 1973).

The general advantages of MRI in medical imaging, especially the acquisition of overlap-free multiplanar images with a high contrast range, are well established. Less well known is the fact that the breast was one of the earliest objects of MRI research. Raymond Damadian suggested in 1971 that it might be possible to differentiate tumors of the breast (Damadian 1971). In 1979 Peter Mansfield published the first MR images of breast tumors (Mansfield et al. 1979). However, neither the subsequent in-vitro test tube studies nor the later in-vivo tissue measurements of T1 and T2 relaxation times allowed reliable differentiation between benign and malignant breast lesions (Ross et al. 1982; El Yousef et al. 1983; Heywang et al. 1985; Kaiser and Zeitler 1985) (Fig. 1.1). For this reason, MR imaging of the breast was not initially widely accepted.

The technical breakthrough in modern MRI of the breast occurred in the mid-1980s with the development of fast gradient-echo imaging sequences with small flip angles, dubbed fast low-angle shot (FLASH), by Jens Frahm and Axel Haase of the Max Planck Institute for Biophysical Chemistry in Göttingen (Frahm et al 1986; Haase et al 1986). The FLASH method enabled fast dynamic imaging and thus the informative use of paramagnetic contrast materials (CM) such as gadolinium chelates. The introduction of specialized surface coils further improved the performance of dynamic, contrast-enhanced (CE) examinations of the breast, so that sufficiently high spatial resolution became possible.

In the following years, MRI of the breast was principally influenced by the research of Sylvia Heywang and Werner Kaiser, resulting in two schools of thought and much debate. Whereas Kaiser, who utilized two-dimensional (2D) FLASH sequences, favored a high temporal resolution, Heywang employed three-dimensional (3D) FLASH sequences favoring a higher spatial resolution. Today, the debate as to which technique yields superior diagnostic results is of only historical interest. MRI examinations of the breast employing modern 3D sequences and present-day scanners with improved gradient performance and power can now provide both high temporal as well as high spatial resolution.

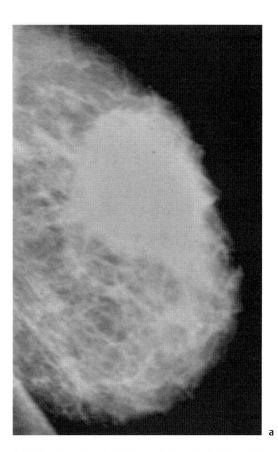

a

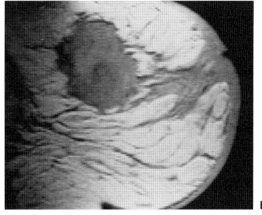

b

Fig. 1.**1 a, b Inflammatory breast cancer.**
a Conventional mammography.
b MRI provides no additional diagnostic information compared with conventional mammography (T1-weighted examination without contrast from 1985).

2 Preparing and Informing the Patient

Before an examination begins, the patient must remove all ferromagnetic items (jewelry, watch, wallet, etc.). All upper-body clothing should be entirely removed and replaced with a gown open to the front.

● General Contraindications for MR Mammography

Because the diagnostic questions that are to be answered by MR mammography are not acutely life-threatening, it is necessary to avoid any possible injury to the patient that could be caused by performing this examination. The following are widely accepted contraindications to MR imaging:

- Cardiac pacemakers
- Heart valves and surgical clips (in heart or brain) made of MR-incompatible materials
- Heart or brain surgery within the previous two weeks
- History of adverse reaction to gadolinium in a previous MR examination using contrast (does not apply to MR examinations of prostheses without contrast medium)

● Obligatory Aspects of Patient Information

- The necessity of administering contrast medium
- Possible intolerance of contrast medium
  (risk of minor adverse reactions, ~1:5000)
  (risk of major adverse reactions, ~1:500 000)
- Written declaration of consent by patient (informed consent form)

● Optional Aspects of Patient Information

- Information about the purpose of the examination
- Information about the length of the examination (10–15 minutes)
- An indication of the expected background noise
- Stress on the necessity of remaining motionless during examination so as to avoid producing movement artifacts
- Advance warning of delivery of contrast and the associated sensations(temporary feeling of coolness in the arm).

● Patient Preparation

- Place a venous access (18–20 gauge) into the cubital or cephalic vein.
- Avoid using the lower arm veins for administration of contrast medium (longer inflow phase).
- Connect extension tubes (1.5 m length, 4 ml volume).
- Allow a short rest period before positioning the patient on the MR table.
- Place the patient in comfortable prone position.
- Apply hearing protection (headset).
- Give a panic bulb to the patient to set off an alarm in case of claustrophobia, nausea, etc.

● Start of Examination

- Notify the patient that the examination will begin.

3 Technique and Methods

Basic Principles of Magnetic Resonance Imaging

Since Paul Lauterbur published his first reports on magnetic resonance imaging (MRI) 30 years ago, it has developed into the mature and versatile imaging technique of today (Lauterbur 1973). The method employs the physical principles of nuclear magnetic resonance (NMR), which have been described by a number of chemists and physicists including Nobel prize winners Isidor Rabi, Edgar Purcell, Felix Bloch, and Richard Ernst. According to the laws of electromagnetism, the rotating motion of an electrically charged particle induces a localized magnetic field around the particle. Certain nuclei—the proton (hydrogen nucleus) and those nuclei possessing an odd number of protons and neutrons, have an intrinsic angular momentum, or *spin*.

For MR imaging, the hydrogen nucleus, or proton, is preferred because of its high concentration in biological tissues (water, fat). In addition to its high abundance, it has the highest magnetic moment of all natural isotopes. In the absence of an external magnetic field, the orientations of the magnetic spins are distributed randomly, so that their magnetic dipoles have no net external effect. When hydrogen nuclei are placed in a strong external magnetic field, these atomic nuclei align themselves with the static magnetic field B_0 in one of two orientations (corresponding to different magnetic quantum numbers): parallel to the field, i.e., „spin up" (the lower-energy state); or antiparallel to the field, i.e., „spin down" (the higher energy state). Because the energy difference between the two states is small, they are almost equally probable. For protons in an applied field of 1.5 T /tesla), the lower-energy state is favored by only one additional proton per 100 000 protons. In addition, because each proton is spinning around its own axis and experiences a torque when exposed to a magnetic field, the spin vectors are forced to gyrate, or *precess* similarly to a spinning top in the earth's gravitational field. This *precessional frequency* ω of the protons' magnetic moments, also called the *Larmor frequency*, is linearly dependent on the magnetic field strength B_0:

$$\omega = \gamma \times B_0$$

The proportionality constant γ is specific for the type of nucleus and is called the *gyromagnetic ratio*. The joint alignment of the spin vectors in the magnetic field creates the macroscopic magnetic moment or *magnetization M*. It is this net magnetic moment that is responsible for the induction of the MR signal in the receiver coil.

A short burst of *radiofrequency* (RF) excitation at the appropriate material-dependent resonant frequency (42 MHz for protons at 1 T) causes a reorientation of the protons' magnetization vector out of the alignment with the longitudinal axis of the magnetic field, i.e., the macroscopic magnetization experiences the torque of the RF field and is forced to rotate about it. The degree of displacement, the *flip angle* α, is dependent on the amplitude and duration of the excitation pulse and is expressed in angular degrees. After the RF pulse is turned off, the protons resume their original positions of longitudinal alignment with the static magnetic field, i.e., they *relax*. During this relaxation process, the energy absorbed by the nuclei is reemitted as RF radiation or is lost through molecular interactions such as electromagnetic dipole–dipole interactions and thermal dissipation. The emitted electromagnetic signal (the MR signal) can be detected as an induced voltage by special receiver coils and translated into an image.

The restoration of the magnetization vector to its original orientation is an exponential process described by the increase of magnetization in the longitudinal plane (*spin–lattice interaction* or *T1 relaxation time*), and the decay of transverse magnetization (*spin–spin interaction* or *T2 relaxation time*). The decay of transverse magnetization is caused by fluctuations of the molecular dipole fields that cause dephasing of the precessing spin vectors. Field inhomogeneities give rise to an additional dephasing of the aligned spins, denoted by adding a star to the relaxation time T2 (T2*). The relaxation times are the times it takes for the RF signal to exponentially rise (T1) or decay (T2) to half its maximum value. Fortunately for the contrast in MR images, T1 and T2 relaxation times are unique for each type of tissue.

For image generation, the emitted signals or RF echoes must be assigned to a specific location on a three-dimensional matrix. Spatial localization is achieved by applying linear magnetic field gradients in *x*, *y*, and *z* directions of space. The spatial encodings for the 2D and 3D techniques are performed differently, however. In the 2D technique, selection of a section is done by simultaneously switching the slice-selection gradient and RF excitation, followed by phase and frequency encoding in-plane. In the 3D technique, a volume is excited with RF and a second phase encoding is performed orthogonally to the first.

The contrast of MR images is influenced by two types of factors: material-specific factors and external factors.

Major material-specific factors include proton density and T1 and T2 relaxation times. External factors include hardware and software parameters (e.g., slice thickness, angulation, number of acquisitions), the type of pulse sequence used (e.g., spin-echo, gradient-echo, fat saturation), the field strength, and whether or not contrast material is administered.

Numerous different pulse sequences can be used for acquiring MR images. Some basic aspects of spin-echo (SE) and gradient-echo (GE) sequences are explained in the following text. GE sequences are especially important for dynamic MR mammography.

In a conventional SE sequence, excitation results from a slice-selective 90° RF pulse, which cancels the longitudinal magnetization and converts it into a transverse magnetization. After half the echo time (TE) has passed, it is followed by a 180° RF pulse, which rephases or refocuses the precessing spins to compensate for signal loss due to inhomogeneities in the magnetic field. Hence, a maximum signal emission, the *spin echo*, will result at the echo time TE. This entire pulse cycle is repeated with a repetition time TR. Depending on the selected echo time and repetition time, the resulting images are T1-weighted, T2- weighted, or proton-weighted.

The echo in GE sequences is produced not by applying a 180° RF pulse but by switching a gradient reversal, causing a refocused RF echo, i.e., gradient echo. In addition, the initial 90° RF pulse can be substituted by a smaller pulse with a flip angle $\alpha < 90°$, which does not use the entire longitudinal magnetization. Although this results in a decreased signal intensity compared to the SE, it allows much faster image generation and acquisition. Compared with SE sequences, GE sequences are more prone to artifacts due to greater sensitivity to field inhomogeneities such as susceptibility differences in tissues (bone, air) or to metal clips. The echo time length, however, also has a major influence. GE sequences are more sensitive to paramagnetic contrast materials.

MRI signal production can be modified by the administration of contrast material. Paramagnetic substances are primarily used for this purpose, but superparamagnetic materials are also administered. Both types of material have the property of changing the relaxation times of the anatomical structures imaged. The major effect of paramagnetic contrast materials is to shorten the T1 relaxation time of the tissues, resulting in signal enhancement. Dynamic MR mammography takes advantage of this effect, which increases signal intensity via increased CM uptake in (neo-)vascularized regions in the T1-weighted sequences. Superparamagnetic substances, which exert a strong shortening effect on T2, are not utilized in MR mammography.

Diagnostic Units

Diagnostic Systems for MR Mammography (Table 3.1)

Table 3.**1**   Diagnostic Units for MR Mammography

General Electric Medical Systems (GE) Co.	
• Signa Horizon LX	1.0 T
• Signa Horizon LX	1.5 T
• Signa MR/i	1.0 T
• Signa MR/i	1.5 T
Philips Co.	
• Gyroscan T5-NT	0.5 T
• Gyroscan T10-NT	1.0 T
• Gyroscan ACT-NT	1.5 T
Siemens Co.	
• Magnetom Symphony	1.5 T
• Magnetom Harmony	1.0 T
• Magnetom Vision and Vision plus	1.5 T
• Magnetom Impact Expert and Expert plus	1.0 T
• Magnetom Impact	1.0 T
• Magnetom 63 SP and SP 4000	1.5 T
• Magnetom 42 SP and 42 SP 4000	1.0 T

Sequence Synonyms (Table 3.2)

Table 3.**2**   Synonyms for Examination Sequences in MR Mammography Used by Different Manufacturers

	GE	Philips	Siemens
Spin-echo	SE	SE	SE
Turbo-spin-echo	FSE	TSE	TSE
Inversion recovery	IR	IR	IR
Inversion recovery FatSat	STIR	STIR	STIR
Gradient-echo, T1-weighted	SPGR	T1-FFE	FLASH
Gradient-echo, T2-weighted	SSFP	T2-FFE	PSIF
Turbo-gradient	FSPGR	T1-TFE	TurboFLASH

Surface Coils

In order to achieve adequate spatial resolution in MR mammography, dedicated surface coils made especially to fit the form of the breast must be used. Commercially available devices that allow a simultaneous bilateral examination are designed for the patient lying prone with both breasts hanging freely in the lumen of the breast coil. Although unilateral breast coils have the advantage of a more homogeneous magnetic field, they have the disadvantage of requiring the patient to return for a second examination on a separate day. For this reason, bilateral breast coils should be used, allowing a single application of CM in a simultaneous MR examination of both breasts (Figs. 3.**1**–3.**3**).

Time of Examination

The circulation in the female breast is subject to hormonal changes. As a result, the CM uptake in the breast varies according to the phase of the menstrual cycle. An intraindividual comparative study on young female test subjects showed that the degree of enhancement of disturbing signals was least in the second week of the menstrual cycle and greatest in the first and fourth weeks (Kuhl et al. 1995). These results were confirmed in studies on perimenopausal and postmenopausal women (Müller-Schimpfle et al. 1997). Although contrast-enhancing patterns typical for malignancy were rarely seen as a result of cyclic fluctuations, appointments for menstruating women should be made accordingly if the reason for referral allows (Fig. 3.**4**).

MR mammography may be performed without limitation after both fine-needle biopsy and large-core biopsy of a breast lesion without significant hematoma. Neither of these procedures results in increased contrast enhancement and they therefore do not interfere with the interpretation of the study (Fischer et al 1996).

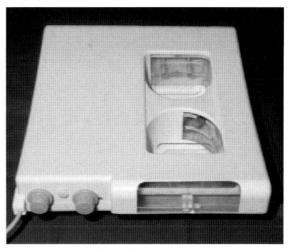

Fig. 3.**1**   **Breast surface coil.**
Siemens Co. surface coil.

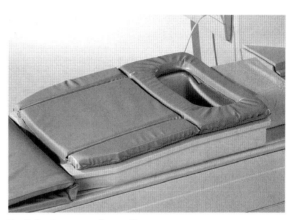

Fig. 3.**2**   **Breast surface coil.**
Philips Co. surface coil.

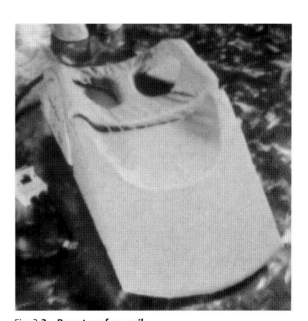

Fig. 3.**3**   **Breast surface coil.**
GE Co. surface coil.

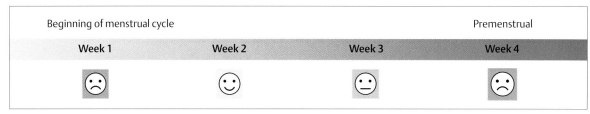

Fig. 3.**4**   **Optimal appointment week for performing MR mammography depending on the menstrual cycle.**

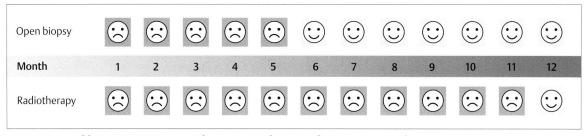

Fig. 3.**5**   **Interval between previous open biopsy or irradiation and MR mammography.**

MR mammography should not be performed within a period of six months after open biopsy so as to avoid problems in interpreting areas of increased enhancement resulting from wound healing. Following lumpectomy with irradiation, this interval is increased to 12 months after completion of radiation therapy (Fig. 3.**5**).

If medical and organizational reasons allow, galactography should not be performed before a planned MR mammography examination; areas of increased enhancement may result in the breast segment examined. If galactography has already been performed, reactive CM enhancement must be considered as a differential diagnosis (see Fig. 6.**13**).

Patient Positioning

In most whole-body scanners, the patient is examined in the prone position with both arms lying flat against the body (Figs.3.**6** and 3.**7**). Alternatively, the arms may be crossed above the head. In this position, however, it may not be possible to place the breasts completely in-

side the breast coil, limiting the examination. After sliding the patient into the magnet bore, it is important to ensure that the extension tubing is accessible beside the patient's feet.

Breast Compression

Adequate breast compression is necessary to reduce motion artifacts during an MR examination. This is especially true for the subtraction technique generally used in Europe. Such artifacts are less disturbing in the primary fat saturation technique.

Numerous approaches have been tried to achieve better compression of the breast inside the coil; wearing a T-shirt during the examination and lateral coil padding are not very promising. More effective approaches use

ventral padding of the breast inside the coil with specialized inserts in different sizes (Fig. 3.**8**). Experience has also been good using a compression device that flattens the breasts in the cranio-caudal (cc) direction (Fig. 3.**9**). This device not only reduces motion artifacts but also decreases the breast thickness in the cc-direction, thereby significantly reducing the slice thickness in the axial MR view (Schorn et al 1998). Newer surface coils with integrated compression devices are

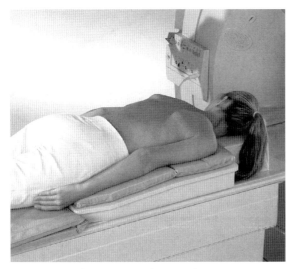

Fig. 3.**6** **Typical positioning of patient for MR mammography.**

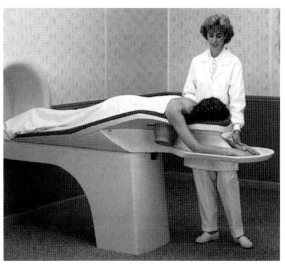

Fig. 3.**7** **Prone positioning of patient in dedicated breast MR unit.**
(Advanced Mammography Systems, Inc.)

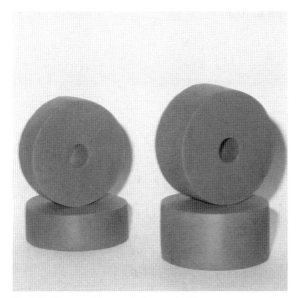

Fig. 3.**8** **Foam rubber pads for ventral breast compression.**

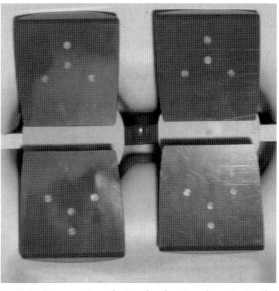

Fig. 3.**9** **Compression device for bracing breasts in the cranio-caudal direction.** View from above.

presently available that compress the breast in the medio-lateral direction. These, however, cause an unfavorable increase of object thickness in axial angulation (Fig. 3.**10**).

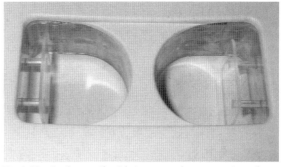

Fig. 3.**10** **Surface coil with integrated compression plates for medio-lateral bracing.**

Field Strength

Presently recommended systems for the performance of MR mammography with contrast material have field strengths of 0.5 T to 1.5 T (tesla). It is not advisable to use systems with a field strength less than 0.5 T for these examinations and most published studies using fast GE sequences have been performed on higher field strength systems (1.0 or 1.5 T). The advantage of 1.0 T and 1.5 T systems over 0.5 T systems is that paramagnetic CM has a greater effect on the signal due to the increased T1 relaxation times of enhancing tissues at higher field strengths (for carcinoma tissue, T1 at 1.5 T = 960 ms; T1 at 1.0 T = 600 ms). However, Kuhl and co-workers have demonstrated that examinations on a 0.5 T system using an adapted pulse sequence in a 3D technique yield very good results. In fact, the overall results of an intraindividual comparative study showed that these results were better than those obtained by examinations on a 1.5 T system using a 2D technique (Fig. 3.**11**). Examinations on both systems were performed with a CM dose of 0.1 mmol Gd-DTPA/kg BW (Kuhl et al. 1995).

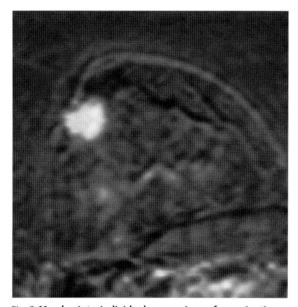
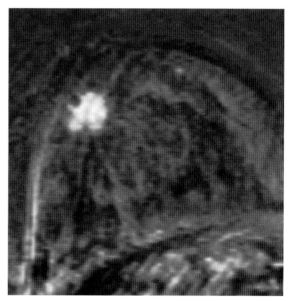

Fig. 3.**11 a, b   Intraindividual comparison of examinations on 0.5 T and 1.5 T systems.**
a Examination using 0.5 T system.

b Examination using 1.5 T system yielding identical image information. (Images provided by the university of Bonn, courtesy of Dr. C.K. Kuhl.)

2D and 3D Techniques

Definition

The **2D technique** in MR mammography is a method in which single axial slices are excited (Fig. 3.**12a**). There should be no gaps between these slices. According to physical principles there is theoretically a signal decrease in the peripheral areas of each slice, but it is not large enough to have any clinical significance.

With an object thickness of ~12 cm, roughly 30 slices with a slice thickness of 4 mm are usually acquired. The field of view (FOV) is rectangular and includes an area within the intrathoracic space. The repetition times (TR) lie in the range of ~200–350 ms, allowing the acquisition of a sufficient number of slices within the TR interval. The ideal flip angle is between 70° and 90°.

In the **3D technique**, the entire breast is excited as a volume (Fig. 3.**12b**). This volume can be divided into so-called *partitions*, or slices of variable thickness, in any desired plane. 3D imaging allows the depiction of thin slices without gaps in a defined slice profile. Generally a volume block of 120 mm with, for example, 30 partitions is used for an examination with axial angulation. The resulting slice thickness is 4 mm. Coronal angulation permits the use of a rectangular FOV. The resulting time gain allows the acquisition of a greater number of partitions, optimizing the spatial resolution (e.g., 60 partitions with a slice thickness of 2 mm). The commonly selected repetition times in the order of 10 ms are shorter than those for the 2D technique. The flip angle is typically 25°.

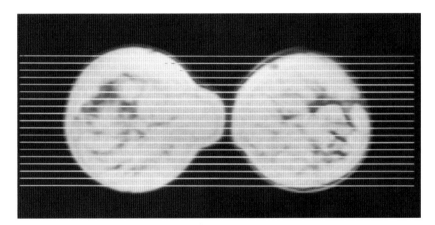

Fig. 3.**12 a, b**   **Comparison of 2D and 3D techniques.**
a   Acquisition of single slices (2D technique).

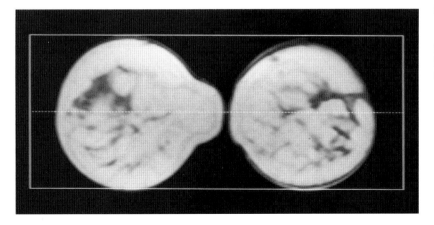

b   Acquisition of a volume block (3D technique).

Both images were generated on the basis of a primary coronal scan slice.

Comparison of the 2D and 3D Techniques

Both the 2D and the 3D techniques may be used without reservation for the contrast-enhanced MR examination of the breast on 1.0 T and 1.5 T systems. A 0.5 T system can also be used successfully in combination with the 3D technique for such examinations (Kuhl et al. 1995).

Both techniques have advantages and disadvantages that do not significantly influence the assessment or predictive value of the MR mammogram. The decision as to which of these techniques to use depends largely on the experience of the examiner. It is therefore not advisable to frequently vary the technique used. In the following, the major advantages of both techniques are compared (Fig. 3.**13**).

- **Advantages of the 2D Technique**

  – Lower susceptibility to artifacts due to single slice acquisition
  – Higher signal efficiency (repetition time ~300 ms)
  – More favorable relationship between the signal curve and CM concentration in the range of diagnostically relevant dosages
  – Lower CM dose (recommended dose 0.1 mmol/kg BW)

- **Advantages of the 3D Technique**

  – Possibility of using coronal angulation with rectangular FOV and consequent reduction of slice thickness (e.g., 2 mm)
  – Option for multiplanar reconstruction
  – Technique of choice for systems with field strength of 0.5 T

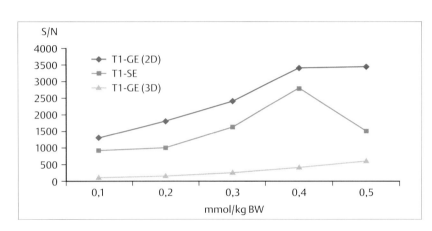

Fig. 3.**13 Signal increase with Gd-DTPA concentration (2D and 3Dtechniques).** Comparison of signal curves for T1-weighted GE sequences in 2D and 3D techniques plotted against CM concentration. A T1-weighted SE sequence is also shown for reference. The diagnostically relevant CM dosage lies between 0.1 and 0.3 mmol/kg BW.

Study Protocols

Tables 3.**3a** and 3.**3b** give examples of protocols for MR mammography uisng the 2D and 3D techniques, respectively (see Fig. 3.**14**).

Table 3.**3a** Protocols for Dynamic MR Mammography (2D Technique)

Parameter	Technique Göttingen[1]	Bonn[2]
Field strength	1.5 T	1.5 T
Gradient field strength	25 mT/m	23 mT/m
Time-to-echo, TE	5 ms	4.6 ms
Time-to-repetition, TR	336 ms	260 ms
Flip angle, α	90°	90°
Field-of-view, FOV	~320 mm	~300 mm
Matrix	256 × 256	256 × 256
Volume slice thickness	—	—
Partitions	—	—
Number of slices	32	31
Single slice thickness	4 mm	3 mm
Sequence time	87 s	55 s
Orientation	Axial	Axial
No. of measurements before CM	1	1
No. of measurements after CM	5	6

[1] Sequence used at the University Hospital, Göttingen
[2] Sequence used at the University Hospital, Bonn (courtesy of Dr. C.K. Kuhl).

Table 3.**3b** Protocols for Dynamic MR Mammography (3D Technique)

Parameter	Technique Halle[1]	Tübingen[2]
Field strength	1.0 T	1.0 T
Gradient field strength	15 mT/m	n.a.
Time-to-echo, TE	6 ms	7 ms
Time-to-repetition, TR	13 ms	14 ms
Flip angle, α	50°	25°
Field-of-view, FOV	160 mm × 320 mm	320 mm
Matrix	100 × 256	179 × 256
Volume slice thickness	160	128
Partitions	64	32
Number of slices	—	—
Single slice thickness	2.5 mm	4 mm
Sequence time	85 s	81 s
Orientation	Coronal	Axial
No. of measurements before CM	1	1
No. of measurements after CM	6	4

[1] Sequence used at the University Hospital, Halle (courtesy of Prof. Dr. S.H. Heywang-Köbrunner).
[2] Sequence used at the University Hospital, Tübingen (courtesy of PD Dr. M. Müller-Schimpfle).

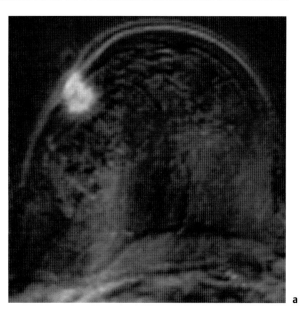

a

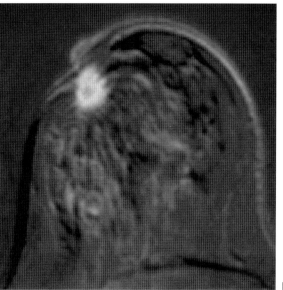

b

Fig. 3.**14a, b Intraindividual comparison of images acquired in 2D and 3D technique. Retromamillary breast cancer.**
a 2D technique.
b 3D technique. Equivalent image quality.

Maximum Protocol (IIBM Study Protocol)

An international multicenter study (12 centers; the International Investigation of Breast MR Imaging) used a so-called *maximum protocol* with respect to spatial and temporal resolution, as well as the administered CM dose. The measurement parameters of this protocol in the 3D technique are presented in Table 3.**4**.

A powerful computer is necessary for the generation and manipulation of the 6 × 64 single images and at least 64 subtraction images that are created by this study protocol. Furthermore, due to the coronal slicing, in which the contrasted veins are seen in cross section and appear as round, lesionlike structures, it is necessary to present and view subtraction images in a maximum-intensity projection (MIP technique; p. 21) (Fig. 3.**15**).

Table 3.**4**   IIBM (International Investigation of Breast MR Imaging) Protocol for Dynamic MR Mammography

Parameter	Field Strength	
	1.0 T	1.5 T
Time-to-repetition, TR	14 ms	12 ms
Time-to-echo, TE	7 ms	5 ms
Flip angle, α	25°	25°
Matrix (rectangular FOV)	96 × 256	102 × 256
Volume slice thickness	160 mm	160 mm
Partitions	64	64
Single slice thickness	2.5 mm	2.5 mm
Sequence time	87 s	87 s
Orientation	Coronal	Coronal
No. of measurements before CM	1	1
No. of measurements after CM	5	6

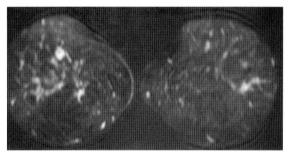 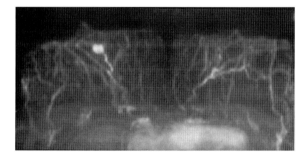

Fig. 3.**15 a, b   Maximum protocol (IIBM).**
a Representative single coronal slice (image subtraction). Depiction of hypervascularized lesion on the right, between the two upper quadrants. In addition, many punctate hypervascularized areas bilaterally.

b Presentation of findings in MIP technique. Imaging of suspicious lesion on the right. Intramammary veins correlate with hypervascularized areas seen in single slices.

Ultrafast Technique

There have been a few attempts to increase the specificity of dynamic MR mammography by ultrafast imaging. In these studies, single slices were taken through lesions that were already obvious in the precontrast images and examinations performed with a very high temporal resolution of 1–2 seconds/sequence. The use of ultrafast contrast-enhanced GE resulted in a specificity of over 80% (Boetes et al. 1994). Our own study investigating this ultrafast technique was not able to verify these findings (Schorn et al. 1998). The inflow of contrast within the tumor was evaluated with respect to the first-pass effect in the aorta. This study showed that an ultrafast technique is not better able to differentiate between hypervascularized malignant and benign tumors than the formerly described techniques (Fig. 3.**16**). At present, sequences that allow such a high temporal resolution only for representative single slices do not increase the specificity of MR mammography.

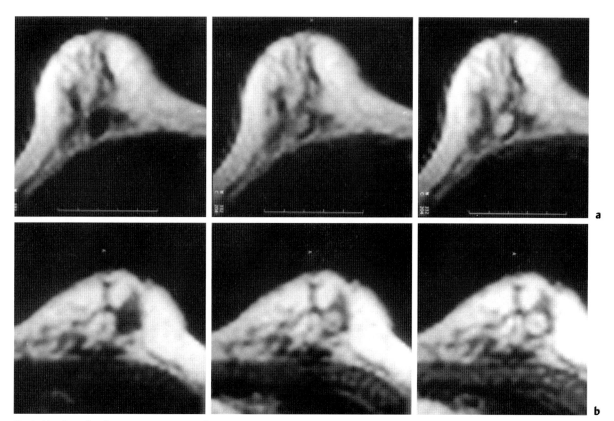

a

b

Fig. 3.16 a, b Ultrafast MR mammography.
a Hypervascularized fibroademona.
b Invasive ductal carcinoma.
  Intraindividual comparison. Identical time delay before CM detection within both lesions, 14 seconds after CM first-pass through the ascending aorta. Images: precontrast, 14 seconds postcontrast, and 22 seconds postcontrast. T1-weighted turbo-FLASH sequence (TR/TE/FA 5.8 ms/3.2 ms/ 8°, slice thickness 6 mm, CM dose 0.1 mmol Gd-DPTA/kg BW at a flow rate of 4 ml/s, sequence length 1 second, reference slice through ascending aorta, temporal resolution 2seconds/sequence) in single slice technique through lesion localized in precontrast image.

High-resolution (HR) Technique

It is possible to increase the spatial resolution by optimizing the matrix (e.g., from a 256 matrix to a 512 matrix), by decreasing the single slice thickness (e.g., from 4 mm to 2 mm), or by selecting a different sequence (e.g., SE sequence instead of GE sequence). All of these changes improve the spatial resolution at the cost of decreasing the temporal resolution. In our experience, therefore, the HR technique should be reserved for nondynamic examinations. These are the optional T2-weighted sequence and the precontrast T1-weighted examination, which can be performed as a high-resolution sequence before acquisition of the dynamic measurement series.

The advantage of the HR technique lies in the more detailed depiction of parenchymal structures in the precontrast examination (Fig. 3.**17**). However, our own studies did not substantiate in advantages the imaging of very small lesions in contrast-enhanced MR examinations. This is due mainly to the increase in signal noise (Fig. 3.**18**).

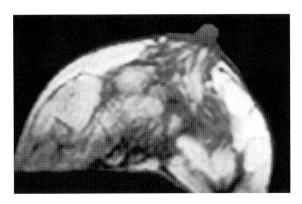
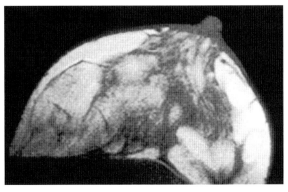

Fig. 3.**17 a, b**   **Intraindividual comparison of HR technique.**
a Sequence with usual spatial resolution: T1-WI, FLASH, slice thickness 4 mm, matrix 256 mm × 256 mm.

b High resolution sequence: T1-WI, FLASH, slice thickness 4 mm, matrix 512 mm × 512 mm. Better detail imaging in HR technique.

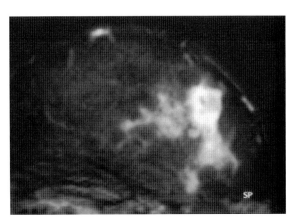
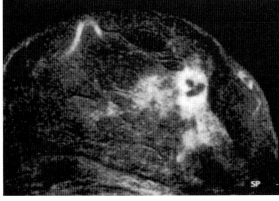

Fig. 3.**18 a, b**   **Intraindividual comparison of HR technique.**
a Sequence with a 256 matrix (subtraction image).

b Sequence with a 512 matrix (subtraction image).
The HR technique shows no advantages in the imaging of peritumoral spreading.

Fat Saturation Techniques

Signal-intense fat tissue can significantly reduce the probability of detecting contrast-enhancing lesions in T1-weighted sequences. This makes it essential to suppress or eliminate the fat signal in such studies. There are two basic means to achieve this:

- Subtraction of identical images before and after contrast
- Generation of primary fat saturation sequences

Image subtraction has become established in Europe as the method of choice for fat suppression; American groups prefer primary fat saturation sequences (Fig. 3.**19**). The *RODEO sequence* (rotating delivery of ex citation off resonance) introduced by S.E. Harms should be mentioned here. In this, frequency-selective saturation of the fat signal is obtained with the combination of a GE sequence and a so-called *magnetization transfer* (MT). Disadvantages of this method are the extremely long acquisition time (~3–5 minutes), which limits the evaluation of hemodynamic characteristics, and occasional inhomogeneous fat suppression.

In most cases fat suppression can be achieved by applying a high-frequency impulse at a shift of 220 Hz just before performing the actual measurements. Saturated fat tissue then emits no signal during the examination. It is generally possible to send such a fat-suppressing impulse before any sequence, but doing so prolongs the examination time. In addition, the RODEO sequence is highly sensitive to inhomogeneities of the main magnetic field. Particularly in MR mammography, the eccentric location of the breasts often prevents homogeneous fat signal suppression.

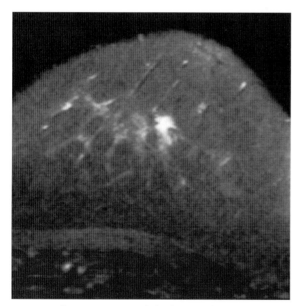 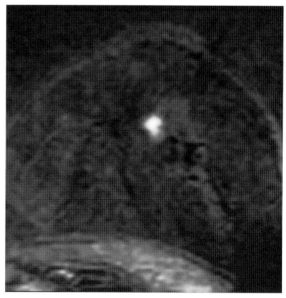

Fig. 3.19 a, b   Suppression of the fat signal in MR mammography.
a Hypervascularized lesion in a primary fat saturation sequence (T1-WI SE sequence, 512 matrix, 3:08 minutes).

b Intraindividual comparison of the same lesion after image subtraction of a T1-WI FLASH sequence (256 matrix, 1:27 min.).

T2-weighted Sequences

In T2-weighted sequences, hydrous or edematous structures emit an intense signal (Fig. 3.**20**). SE or turbo-spin-echo (TSE) sequences are the T2-weighted sequences most commonly used in MR mammography. Alternatively, inversion recovery (IR) sequences may also be used. T2-weighted images are generally acquired before performing contrast enhanced dynamic measurements.

T2-weighted sequences make it possible to recognize small cysts only a few millimeters in diameter with high sensitivity. In addition, they provide a useful criterion for the differential diagnosis of smooth-bordered hyper-

vascularized lesions: *myxoid fibroadenomas*. These often show a very high CM uptake due to their histology, with only a small degree of fibrosis. In the T2-weighted images, these lesions typically emit a very intense signal, sometimes as pronounced as the signal emitted by cysts. In contrast, carcinomas usually show a much lower signal intensity, similar to or lower than that of normal breast parenchyma; however, T2-weighted sequences play no role in the detection of malignant tumors.

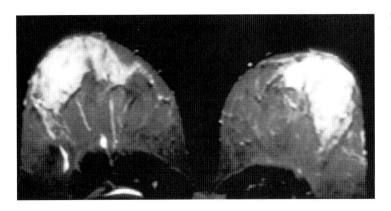

Fig. 3.**20**   **T2-weighted image.**
Normal findings. Signal-intense imaging of edematous parenchyma in a young woman (IR sequence).

Temporal Resolution

In most cases, hypervascularized tumors of the breast show a faster CM uptake than the normal surrounding parenchyma. This is especially true for invasive carcinomas whose maximum signal increase is reached on the average three minutes after CM administration. The signal of breast parenchyma, on the other hand, increases continually during the examination period of 8–10 minutes (Fischer et al. 1993).

The range of variation for signal intensity is great, however, and some carcinomas reach their signal maximum in the first minute after CM administration in the form of a peak with a following wash out phenomenon. Within normal healthy parenchyma there may also be areas of early, intense CM uptake (e.g., adenosis, hormone stimulation), which can cause an early masking of pathological processes (Fig. 3.**21**).

For these reasons, the generally accepted guidelines require that dynamic measurements (at least five measurements after CM administration) have a temporal resolution of 1–2 minutes per sequence. This makes possible the discrimination between pathological processes and surrounding parenchyma, as well as the acquisition of a sufficiently accurate dynamic curve. Semidynamic measurements (e.g., two measurements after CM administration, sequence length ca. five minutes) do not meet these requirements. However, further optimization of the temporal resolution with measurements in the range of seconds does not result in additional advantages (Schorn et al. 1999).

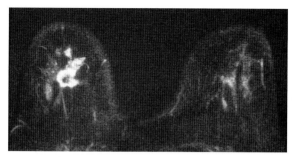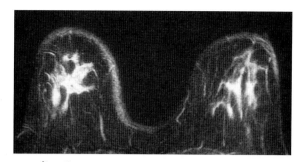

Fig. 3.**21 a, b   Temporal discrimination between tumor and surrounding tissue.**

a Subtraction of the precontrast image from the first measurement after CM administration. Imaging of a carcinoma in the right breast with typical ring enhancement and multifocal tumor spread.

b Masking of these findings in the subtraction of the precontrast image from the second measurement after CM administration due to the rapid CM uptake of the surrounding breast parenchyma. Acquisition time per measurement sequence: 87 seconds.

Spatial Resolution

The spatial resolution of MR mammography is influenced by various factors and adjustment parameters. In particular these are the matrix, dependent upon the chosen FOV, the slice thickness, and the size of the imaged volume.

Examinations performed with axial angulation have a FOV predetermined by the patients' proportions. It is square in shape and generally between 300 and 350 mm in side length. Examinations performed with coronal angulation and 3D technique allow the selection of a rectangular FOV, reducing the slice thickness by 50 %.

The image volume is determined by the requirement that, for diagnostic purposes, both breasts be completely examined. Compression in the craniocaudal orientation can reduce the object thickness by approximately one-third (Schorn et al. 1996).

The matrix normally used is 256 × 256 pixels. Although it is possible to increase it to 512 × 512 pixels, this results in an unacceptable lengthening of the acquisition time to over two minutes using the currently available MR systems.

It is recommended that the selected slice thickness be 2–4 mm. This ensures that tumors with a diameter over 4–8 mm are completely imaged in at least one slice (Fig. 3.**22**).

In general, optimizing the spatial resolution results in a reduction of the temporal resolution. Routine examinations are therefore a compromise between these two characteristics. Notwithstanding this, studies are being performed to evaluate how the predictive value of MR mammography can be improved using protocols with maximal spatial resolution (e.g., $1 \times 1 \times 1\,mm^3$, 3 minutes) or maximal temporal resolution ($3 \times 3 \times 8\,mm^3$, 2.3 seconds).

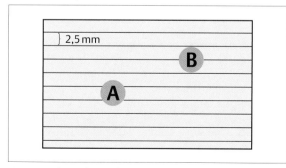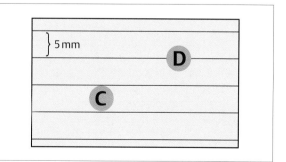

Fig. 3.**22 a, b   Relation between slice thickness and tumor size.**

a When the tumor diameter is greater than or equal to twice the slice thickness, the lesion will always be seen in at least one slice without a partial volume effect (lesions A and B).

b When the tumor diameter lies between one and two times the slice thickness, this is not necessarily the case (lesion D).

Slice Orientation

In principle, it is possible to perform MRI examinations at any angulation. For dynamic MR mammography, the axial and coronal slice orientations are generally preferred. The advantages and disadvantages of these, as well as of the sagittal slice orientation are discussed in the following.

The main advantage of the axial slice orientation is that it makes a good assessment of breast areas near the chest wall possible because partial volume effects between breast tissue and the pectoral muscle (i.e., bony thorax) do not produce ambiguous structures. In addition, intramammary veins are usually imaged along their course, so that they can be recognized as tubular structures and will not be mistaken for round lesions. The main disadvantage of the axial slice orientation is the limited assessment it permits of parenchymal structures in the axillary region, due to cardiac artifacts caused by the phased encoding gradients.

The coronal slice orientation permits the selection of a rectangular FOV, which makes allows reduction of the slice thickness and the optimization of the spatial resolution to ∼2 mm. In addition, artifact-free imaging of parenchymal structures in the axillary tail can be achieved. The disadvantages are that veins are seen in cross section and may be misinterpreted as small, suspicious lesions (Fig. 3.**23**). For this reason it is necessary to postprocess images in MIP technique.

The sagittal slice orientation is not recommended for use in the diagnostic work-up for breast cancer. It is, however, employed in the examinations of prostheses when complications are suspected.

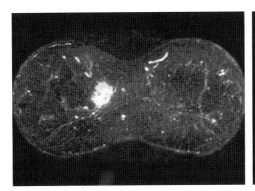 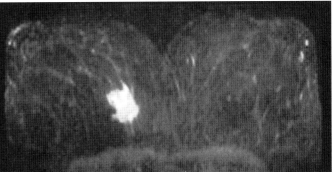

Fig. 3.**23 a, b   Comparison of coronal and axial slice orientations.**
a Hypervascularized lesion in the coronal view (3D sequence). Veins in cross section simulate small, hypervascularized lesions.
b Same lesion in axial reconstruction.

Paramagnetic Contrast Materials

The distinguishing characteristic of a paramagnetic substance is that it has at least one unpaired electron. This electron has a magnetic moment that is ∼1000 times stronger than that of a proton. It is this characteristic that effects a shortening of the T1 and T2 relaxation times. With the T1-weighted sequences used in dynamic MR mammography, an increase in the signal intensity results.

Intravenous administration of an extracellular paramagnetic CM provides a means for imaging the circulatory situation in the breast. Repetitive measurements after CM administration in the form of a semidynamic technique (e.g., two measurements after CM administration) or a dynamic technique (more than two measurements after CM administration) can provide information about the time course of CM uptake and wash-out.

The greatest experience with contrast material in MR mammography is with gadolinium-DTPA (Gd-DTPA). Its chemical structure comprises a Gd-ion with a triple positive charge combined with a DTPA (pentetic acid) derivative, forming a very stable complex (effective stability constant $K_{eff} = 10^{18.3}$ at pH 7.4). No free Gd-atoms have been observed under physiological conditions (Weinmann 1997). In European countries, Gd-DTPA (Magnevist, Schering Co.) is the most commonly used contrast material in MR mammography. Other paramagnetic gadolinium substances are used for contrast enhanced MR mammography in other countries; these include Gd-DOTA, Gadoterate-Meglumine (Dotarem,

Guerbert Co.), Gd-HP-DO3A Gadoteridol (ProHance, Bracco-Byk Gulden Co.), and Gd-DTPA-BMA, Gadodiamide (Omniscan, Nykomed Co.).

Dosage

The recommended contrast dosage for dynamic MR mammography (1.0 and 1.5 T) in 2D technique is 0.1 mmol Gd-DTPA/kg BW. There are reports of advantages in using a higher dosage between 0.15 and 0.2 mmol Gd-DTPA/kg BW for the 3D technique (Heywang-Köbrunner et al. 1994). It is important to remember that the threshold values for the evaluation of contrast-enhancing lesions are dose-dependent and must be adapted accordingly (Fig. 3.**24**).

Mode of Administration

Administration of CM should be either manual or mechanical, into the previously placed cubital venous access, at a rate of 2–3 ml/s. Use of a venous access in the lower arm and hand veins should be avoided. Immediately after CM administration, 20 ml or more of 0.9 % NaCl should be administered to flush out any remainder.

Elimination

Gadolinium-DTPA is eliminated rapidly and completely by renal excretion without tubular reabsorption. The half-time of Gd-DTPA in blood is ~90 minutes. More than 91 % of the administered dose is eliminated after 24 hours.

Tolerance and Adverse Effects

Gadolinium-DTPA is very well tolerated by most patients. From experience with its use in over 20 million examinations, it is estimated to have an adverse reaction rate of under 2 %, of which 80 % are minor reactions.

These minor adverse reactions include nausea, vomiting, allergylike skin and mucous membrane reactions, and local sensations of pain or warmth. It is still necessary to inform the patient of these possibilities and obtain a signed consent form before beginning the examination. Emergency measures to be taken in the case of a major adverse reaction are the same as those for adverse reactions to x-ray CM.

Gd-DTPA in Pregnancy

The absolute safety of Gd-DTPA administration in pregnancy has not yet been proven. Dynamic MR mammography should therefore not be performed on pregnant women.

Gd-DTPA during Lactation

Approximately 0.011 % of the contrast material administered intravenously is eliminated in the breast milk of lactating women. Only ~2 % of this is absorbed by the gastrointestinal tract of a breast-fed child. It is calculated that the plasma concentration of Gd-DTPA for a child weighing 3 kg is 1/1000 of the mothers' plasma concentration. Nevertheless, it is generally recommended that breast feeding be interrupted for 24 hours after administration of CM.

Gd-DTPA and Renal Insufficiency

The elimination of Gd-DTPA depends only upon the glomerular filtration rate. Renal insufficiency is not a contraindication for CM administration. It is recommended, however, that dialysis be performed after the examination if the creatinine clearance in lower than 20 ml/min or the serum creatinine concentration is greater than 3–4 mg/100 ml.

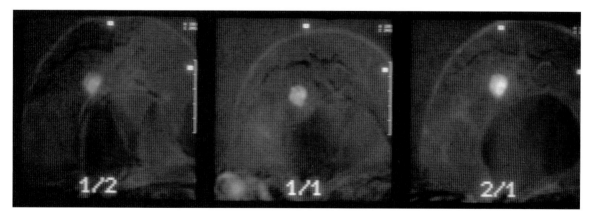

Fig. 3.**24 Intraindividual comparison of the effect of CM dose on the imaging of a hypervascularized fibroadenoma (2D technique).** Image subtraction after intravenous. administration of 0.05, 0.1, and 0.2 mmol Gd-DTPA/kg BW.

Image Postprocessing

The great number of images acquired in dynamic MR mammography makes postprocessing necessary. This serves to detect enhancing lesions, determine the probability of malignancy, and improve the presentation of findings (Fig. 3.**25**).

Image Subtraction

Subtraction of images of identical slices is performed to eliminate the intense fat signal and improve the detection of hypervascularized lesions. Normally, the precontrast image series is subtracted from an early postcontrast image series (first or second series after CM administration) on a pixel-by-pixel basis. Subtraction from later postcontrast image series has not proven useful because the increasing enhancement of healthy breast tissue leads to a masking of suspicious lesions.

Signal–Time Analysis of Enhancing Lesions

The analysis of signal–time curves within representative areas of enhancing lesions allows a further differentiation with respect to the probability of malignancy. The corresponding region of interest (ROI) should be selected such that it includes the greatest possible portion of maximally enhancing area while disregarding less vascularized tumor areas (e.g., central necrotic portions). The size of the ROI should be between two and

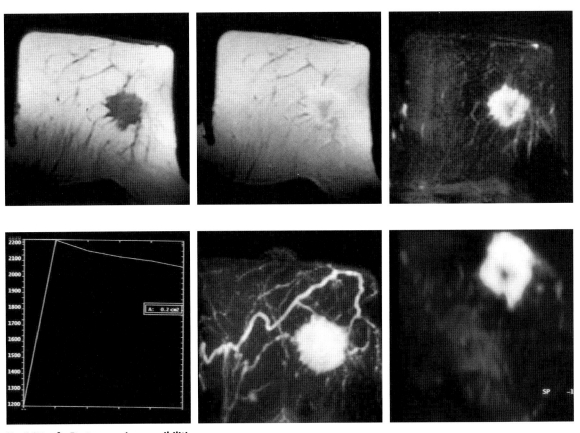

Fig. 3.**25 a–f   Postprocessing possibilities.**
a Precontrast image of breast cancer in a T1-weighted GE sequence.
b Documentation of the lesion in the second postcontrast measurement. Strong enhancement within the tumor reaching the signal intensity of fat tissue.
c Subtraction of the precontrast image from an early postcontrast image (second postcontrast image). Note positioning of the ROI in an area of maximal enhancement within the tumor (here in peripheral ring enhancement).

d Calculation and presentation of signal–time curve corresponding to the ROI of (c).
e MIP image portraying tumor spread and position. **Note**: Ring enhancement seen in single slice is missing due to summation of all slices in this technique.
f Imaging of tumor after multiplanar reconstruction (MPR) of subtracted single slices; for example, to document the relationship of the tumor to the skin (skin involvement).

five pixels. The results of the signal–time analysis can be represented in a numerical fashion with respect to time and, if desired, expressed in terms of a percent increase over the initial values.

Maximum Intensity Projection (MIP)

The MIP technique yields a three-dimensional comprehensive view of both breasts. Based on postprocessed subtraction images in which only image pixels having at least a certain signal intensity are taken into account (threshold value algorithm), the representation of image information gives the impression of a transparent breast that can be viewed from different angles. This form of imaging allows a simpler spatial orientation and is especially suitable for the presentation of suspicious findings. Normally, the MIP technique does not provide additional diagnostically relevant information.

Multiplanar Reconstruction (MPR)

MPR images allow three-dimensional views of partial volumes within the breast. These are also based on postprocessed subtraction images. In special cases, these calrify the topographic relationship between a suspicious lesion and defined anatomical structures (e.g., mammillary region). The MPR technique is seldom used in MR mammography. Like MIP, this technique does not normally provide additional diagnostically relevant information.

Automated Image Postprocessing and Analysis

Various models for computer-aided analysis of dynamic MR examinations of the breast have been published (Figs. 3.**26** and 3.**27**) (Kuhl et al. 1996; Teubner et al. 1995; Knopp et al. 1995). These range from color-coded parameter images, automatically defined ROI's, and cine sequences with repeat rates of 1–2 seconds, to the use of pharmacokinetic models. To date, however, there are no large-scale studies defining the value of these postprocessing and analysis modalities.

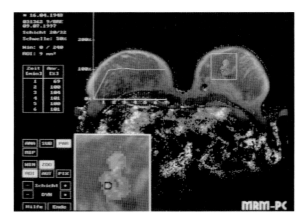

Fig. 3.26 Computer-aided analysis of MR mammography. Documentation of a computer-aided analysis of MR mammography with identification of a hypervascularized lesion on the left (threshold > 50% signal increase). Presentation of signal–time curve including numerical values for the percent signal increase (software, Bieling Co., Bonn, Germany).

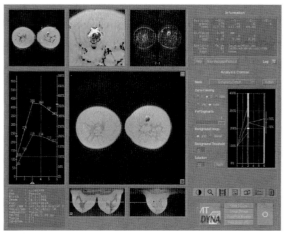

Fig. 3.27 Computer-aided analysis of MR mammography. Documentation of a computer aided analysis of MR mammography with identification of a hypervascularized lesion on the left. Presentation of several signal–time curves, as well as imaging in different views before and after contrast administration (software, MeVis Co., Bremen, Germany).

4 Tumor Angiogenesis
U. Brinck

Basic Principles

The formation of new blood vessels (neoangiogenesis) in breast cancers is functionally important in tumor growth and in blood-borne tumor dissemination. It is also significant in the spread of tumor to the regional lymph nodes. Newly formed blood vessels initially have permeable intercellular connections between the endothelial cells that enable the passage of proteins (and contrast material) into the extravascular space. Neoangiogenesis is initiated in the immediate extraductal surroundings of in-situ carcinomas.

Neoangiogenesis facilitates the metastatic spread of invasive carcinomas since tumor cells can invade newly formed capillaries more easily than preexisting blood vessels. The likelihood of regional lymph node involvement and distant metastases increases with blood vessel density. In contrast to normal local capillaries, new ones have a discontinuous basement membrane. Invasion of capillaries with a discontinuous basement membrane occurs more easily because collagen type IV-specific collagenase is not needed to dissolve it. Neoangiogenesis tends to take place in the immediate vicinity of carcinoma cells because of the chemotactic factors they produce. Tumor cells can therefore invade newly formed capillaries without having to migrate long distances.

The formal process of angiogenesis, originating from preexisting blood vessels, is made up of the following steps:

- Proteolytic breakdown of the basement membrane of preexisting blood vessels as a prerequisite for the formation of new blood vessel sprouts
- Migration of endothelial cells toward an angiogenic (chemotactic) stimulus
- Proliferation of endothelial cells directly behind the front row of migrating cells
- Differentiation of endothelial cells with development of a new vessel lumen

Tumor angiogenesis is modulated by the balance of angiogenesis-promoting factors and angiogenesis inhibitors. These are produced by the tumor cells themselves, or by tumor-associated tissues. Two especially important angiogenesis-promoting factors, produced by the tumor cells, are the basic fibroblast growth factor (bFGF) and the vascular endothelial growth factor (VEGF). Both bind specific receptors on the endothelial cells.

The therapeutic application of angiogenetic inhibitors in the treatment of metastatic disease is currently under study. All have in common that they specifically influence one or more steps in the process of angiogenesis (proteolytic activity, chemotaxis, migration, proliferation of endothelium).

Tumor Angiogenesis and MR Mammography

U. Brinck

Various research groups have endeavored to quantify the extent of tumor angiogenesis by means of immuno-histochemical labeling, and to correlate it with the signal behavior in dynamic MR mammography (Fig. 4.**1**). Early reports were based on immunohistochemical detection of actin and factor VIII-associated antigen (Folkman and Klagsbrunn 1987; Weidner et al. 1991, 1992). In our own series of experiments, we showed that the use of antibodies of the cluster designation (CD) system produced better results. Among the antibodies specific for CD34, the monoclonal mouse antibodies NCL-END, which labels endothelial cells, proved to be very sensitive (Fischer 1998).

In patients with breast cancer, Buadu found a correlation between ring enhancement in MR mammography and the pattern of blood vessel distribution—a high number of blood vessels in the periphery detected by CD34-immunolabeling and a low number of blood vessels in the tumor's fibrotic or necrotic center (Buadu et al. 1997). In another semiquatitative comparative study, he had previously demonstrated a correlation between blood vessel density and the steepness of the initial signal increase ($r = 0.83, P < 0.001$) (Buadu et al. 1996). The high correlation between early CM uptake in MR mammography and the immunohistochemical demonstration of high blood vessel density has been confirmed by other authors (Frouge et al. 1994; Hulka et al. 1997; Siewert et al. 1997). Our own studies, however, did not find such a good correlation. Our comparative CD34 labeling studies showed only a moderate correlation ($r = 0.43, P < 0.001$) with the initial signal increase (Fischer 1998).

Although published data differ on the correlation between the immunohistochemically assessed micro-circulatory status and the signal increase in dynamic MR mammography, blood vessel density is a meaningful factor in this context. Other factors related to signal behavior are changes in blood vessel permeability and the tumor matrix (Brinck et al. 1995). The tumor matrix can consist of fibrotic or necrotic areas, both of which reduce the CM uptake.

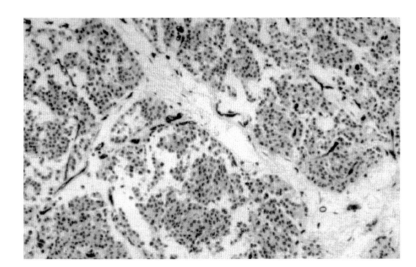

Fig. 4.**1   Immunohistochemical blood vessel labeling (CD34).**
Immunohistochemical demonstration of numerous CD34-positive tumor blood vessels in breast carcinoma.

5 Diagnostic Criteria

Precontrast Examination

The T1-weighted precontrast examination and the optional, complementary T2-weighted measurements permit a specific diagnosis in cases with a typical constellation of findings. In the following, a few typical combinations of findings are presented (Table 5.1, Fig. 5.1).

However, breast cancer cannot be reliably detected and benign and malignant tumors cannot be adequately differentiated without the intravenous administration of contrast.

Table 5.1 Typical Finding Constellations in Specific Lesions

Substrate	T1-weighted Signal	T2-weighted Signal	Lesion
Water	Intermediate	Increased	Cyst
Oil, fat	Increased	Intermediate	Traumatic oil cyst, lipoma, fatty lymph node, fresh hematoma
Acute blood	Decreased	Decreased	Acute hematoma
Old blood	Increased (circular)	Increased	Subacute hematoma
Calcification	Decreased	Decreased	Fibroadenoma, fat necrosis
Metal fragments	Lossed	Lossed	Foreign body
Metal abrasions	Lossed	Lossed	Postoperative finding

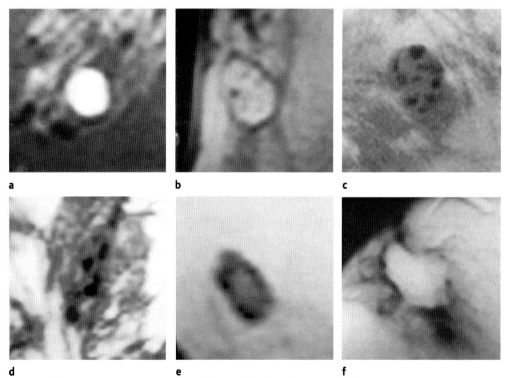

a

b

c

d

e

f

Fig. 5.1 a–f **Precontrast examinations with typical findings for a specific diagnosis.**

a Increased signal intensity in T2-weighted image. Cyst.
b Increased signal intensity in T1-weighted image. Traumatic oil cyst.
c Small endotumoral signal attenuations in T1-weighted image. Fibrotic fibroadenoma with macrocalcifications.

d Localized signal loss in T1-weighted image. Metal abrasions left after operation with electrocauterization.
e Fat equivalent signal in T1-weighted image. Lymph node with fatty changes.
f Increased signal intensity in T1-weighted image. Subacute hematoma after dog bite.

Contrast-enhanced T1-weighted Examinations

Morphology

Form

The form describes the shape of a contrast-enhancing region (Fig. 5.**2**).

Form of contrast-enhancing region
- Round
- Oval
- Polygonal
- Linear
- Branched
- Spiculated

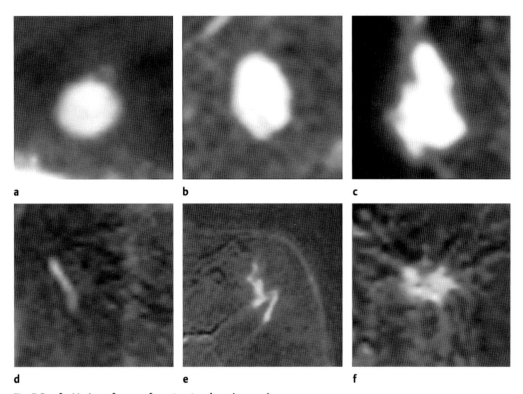

a   b   c

d   e   f

Fig. 5.2 a–f   Various forms of contrast-enhancing regions.
Subtraction images illustrating the various forms of contrast-enhancing regions.
a Round   **d** Linear
b Oval   **e** Branching
c Polygonal   **f** Spiculated

Margins

The margins describe the outer contours of a contrast-enhancing region (Fig. 5.**3**).

Margins of contrast enhancing region
- Well-defined
- Indistinct (ill-defined)

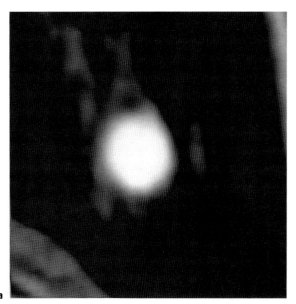
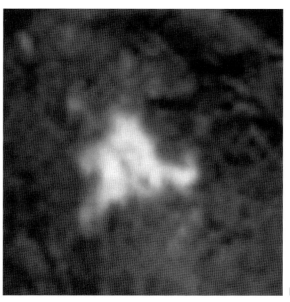

a   **b**

Fig. 5.**3 a, b   Margins of contrast-enhancing region.**
Subtraction images illustrating margin differences.

a Well-defined
b Indistinct.

Pattern

The contrast enhancement pattern describes the spacial distribution of contrast within the contrast-enhancing region (Fig. 5.**4**).

Pattern of contrast enhancing region
- Homogenous
- Inhomogenous
- Septated
- Peripheral (so-called ring-enhancement or rim sign).*

* **Ring-enhancement:** stronger contrast uptake in tumor periphery in comparison to tumor center. (Signal loss in tumor center = necrosis; signal attenuation in tumor center = fibrosis.)

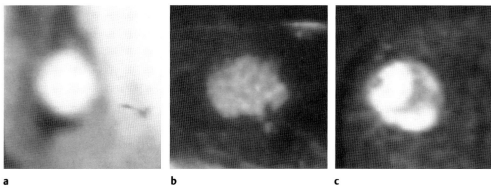

a   **b**   **c**

Fig. 5.**4 a–f   Contrast-enhancement pattern.**
Subtraction images illustrating different contrast-enhancement patterns.

a Homogenous
b Inhomogenous
c Septated

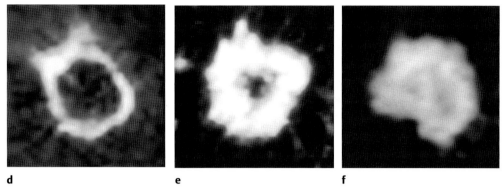

d   **e**   **f**

Fig. 5.**4 d–f**   Examples of so-called ring-enhancement.

Kinetics

Contrast kinetics is the temporal distribution of contrast material during an examination (Fig. 5.**5**).

Benign lesions (e.g., fibroadenomas) usually display a centrifugal CM distribution. An unchanging distribution is unspecific. A centripetal CM spread presupposes a primary ring-enhancement and is therefore normally found in carcinomas.

Kinetics of contrast distribution
• Centrifugal (blooming)
• Unchanging
• Centripetal

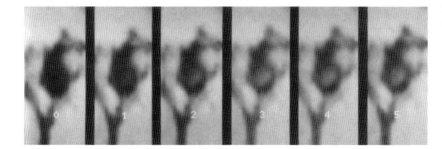

Fig. 5.**5 a, b   Contrast kinetics.**
a Size increase of contrast-enhancing lesion (centrifugal).

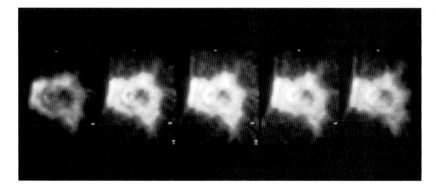

b Centripetal contrast spread after primary enhancement in peripheral regions of the lesion.

Dynamics

Initial Signal Increase

Enhancement dynamics describes the signal intensity changes occurring in a contrast-enhancing region with respect to time. One distinguishes between the initial phase (1–3 minutes after CM administration) and the postinitial phase (3–8 minutes after CM administration). The initial signal increase (in %) is the maximum signal intensity within the first three minutes after CM administration compared to the signal intensity of the precontrast image (Fig. 5.6). It is calculated using the following formula:

Initial signal increase [%] =
$[(\text{Signal}_{\text{post-CM}} - \text{Signal}_{\text{pre-CM}})/\text{Signal}_{\text{pre-CM}}] \times 100$ [%]

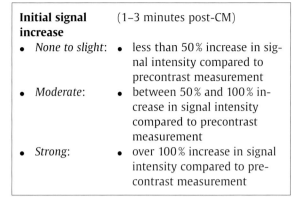

Initial signal increase	(1–3 minutes post-CM)
• *None to slight*:	• less than 50% increase in signal intensity compared to precontrast measurement
• *Moderate*:	• between 50% and 100% increase in signal intensity compared to precontrast measurement
• *Strong*:	• over 100% increase in signal intensity compared to precontrast measurement

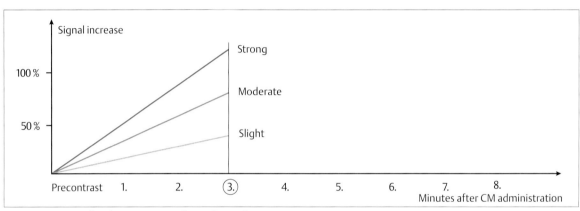

Fig. 5.**6**   **Diagram for determination of initial signal increase.**

Postinitial Signal Behavior

The postinitial signal behavior describes the course of the signal curve between 3 and 8 minutes after contrast administration (Fig. 5.**7**). The signal intensity value after 8 minutes is expressed in relation to the maximum value in the initial phase as follows:

Postinitial signal behavior =
$[(Signal_{8\ min} - Signal_{MAX\ 1-3\ min})/Signal_{MAX\ 1-3.min}] \times 100\ [\%]$

Postinitial signal behavior	(3–8 minutes post-CM)
• Continuous increase:	• signal increase over 10%
• Plateau:	• constant signal intensity (± 10%)
• Wash-out:	• signal decrease over 10%

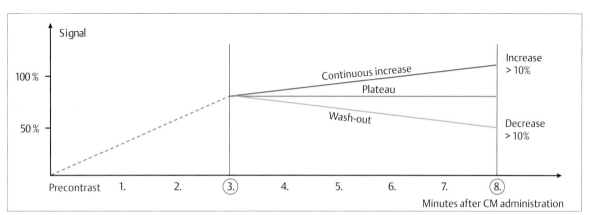

Fig. 5.**7**   **Diagram for determination of postinitial signal behavior.**

Criteria of Malignancy

Table 5.**2** lists criteria in contrast-enhancing MR mammography that strongly indicate the presence of malignancy or are unspecific.

Unifactorial evaluation protocols that take only one threshold parameter into consideration (e.g., signal increase > 90% in the first minute after CM administration, or increase in normalized units > 500) have a significantly lower specificity at an equivalent sensitivity than do multifactorial evaluation protocols (Table 5.**3**).

Table 5.**2** Morphological and Dynamic Criteria for Differentiation between Malignant and Benign Lesions in Contrast-enhanced MR Mammography

Criterion	Suspicious for Malignancy	Unspecific
Form	Branching, spiculated	Round
Margins	Indistinct	Well-defined
Pattern	Ring-enhancement	Inhomogenous
Kinetics	Centripetal	Unchanging
Dynamics (initial)	Strong increase	Moderate increase
Dynamics (postinitial)	Wash-out	Plateau

Table 5.**3** Comparison of Unifactorial and Multifactorial Evaluation Protocols (author's studies)

Protocol	Sensitivity	Specificity	Accuracy
Unifactorial			
Threshold > 90%	96%	31%	78%
Threshold > 500 NU	98%	27%	86%
Multifactorial			
Initial signal increase + postinitial signal + CM distribution + margin definition	98%	59%	87%

NU, normalized unit

Evaluation Score

It is very helpful for the evaluation of lesions to use a multifactorial protocol in which each evaluation criterion receives a point value. Using the system presented in Table 5.**4**, findings with a total score of less than 3 points generally correspond to benign lesions, whereas a total score greater than 3 points indicates malignancy (Fig. 5.**8**). Such a scoring system facilitates the differentiation of contrast-enhancing lesions in MR mammography (Figs. 5.**9**–5.**11**).

Clinical, mammographic, and ultrasonographic findings must always be integrated in the overall evaluation of a lesion (see Chapter 12).

Table 5.**4** Multifactorial Evaluation Protocol

	Criterion		Points
1	Form:	Round	0
		Oval	0
		Polygonal	0
		Linear	0
		Branching	1
		Spiculated	1
2	Margins:	Well-defined	0
		Indistinct	1
3	Enhancing pattern:	Homogenous	0
		Inhomogenous	1
		Septated	0
		Ring-enhancement	2

	Dynamics		
4	Initial signal increase:	< 50%	0
		50–100%	1
		> 100%	2
5	Postinitial signal course:	Steady increase	0
		Plateau	1
		Wash-out	2

Fig. 5.8 Evaluation scores.
Each evaluation criterion can be given a maximum of 1 point (factors 1 and 2 in Table 5.**4**) or 2 points (factors 3–5 in Table 5.**4**). A maximum total score of 8 is possible. The total number of points defines the MRM-BIRADS.

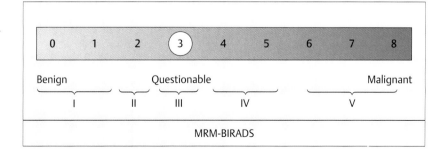

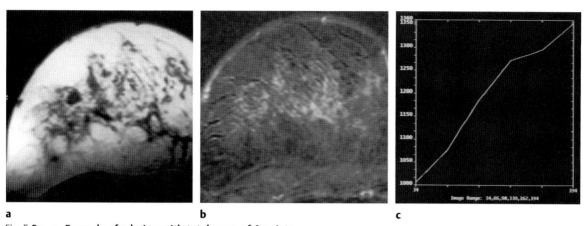

a   b   c

Fig. 5.**9 a–c**   **Example of a lesion with total score of 0 points.**
Round (score 0), well-defined (score 0) lesion; initial signal increase under 20% (sscore 0), postinitial continuous signal increase (score 0).

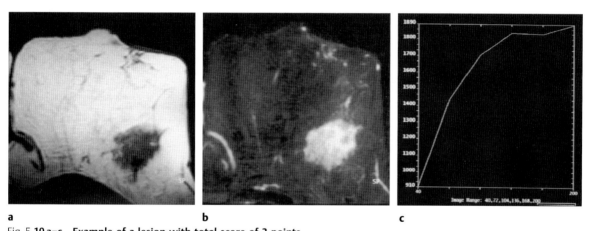

a   b   c

Fig. 5.**10 a–c**   **Example of a lesion with total score of 3 points.**
Oval (score 0) lesion with inhomogenous enhancement (score 1) and partially indistinct margins (score 1). Initial signal increase of ~85% (score 1), postinitial continuous signal increase (score 0).

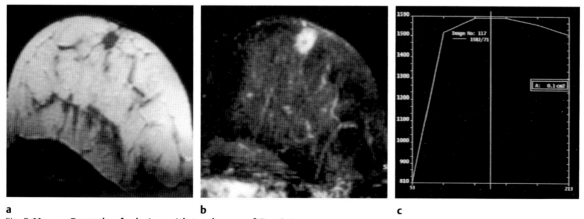

a   b   c

Fig. 5.**11 a–c**   **Example of a lesion with total score of 5 points.**
Oval (score 0) lesion with indistinct margins (score 1). Ring-enhancement (score 2). Initial signal increase of 96% (score 1) with postinitial plateau (score 1).

6 Artifacts and Sources of Error

Incorrect Positioning

The patient to be examined is typically placed in the prone position. The breasts hang in the special breast coil. It is important to take care that all areas of the breast hang freely and completely in the coil lumen, and not outside its sensitive volume (Fig. 6.1). The complete imaging of the breast within the breast coil lumen should always be assured before beginning dynamic measurements. The T2-weighted sequence performed before the dynamic examination is well suited for this purpose and can easily be repeated if inadequate positioning must be corrected.

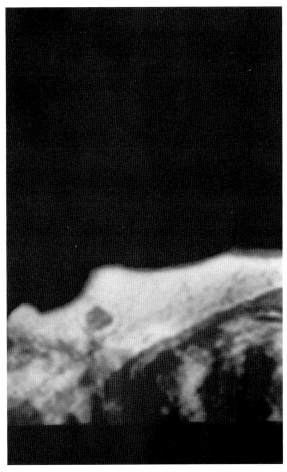

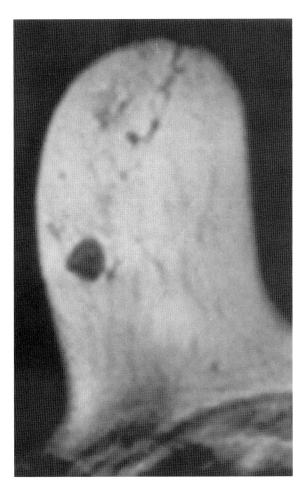

Fig. 6.**1 a, b   Incorrect positioning.**

a Incorrect positioning of the breast inside the surface coil. Hypointense lesion (T1-weighted precontrast study) lies within surrounding fatty tissue at the outer rim of the coil and is overlapped by interfering cardiac artifacts.

b Repeat examination after correct positioning of the breast. Proper imaging of the lesion inside the breast coil lumen.

Improper Administration of Contrast

The paravenous injection of CM can remain undetected if only the precontrast and subtraction images are evaluated; in particular, the subtraction images will simulate normal findings in this case (Fig. 6.**2**). For this reason, it is necessary to ensure correct intravasal administration of contrast by detecting strong enhancement in a typical reference point (e.g., intramammary veins, or internal mammary artery).

Failure to administer a normal saline injection after contrast administration leads to a significant under-

dosage of CM since 4 ml will then remain in the extension tubing. For a woman with a body weight of 70 kg and a desired dosage of 0.1 mmol Gd-DTPA/kg BW, this volume that is not administered amounts to a 30% reduction of the effective dose. Since this affects the signal curves and may result in misinterpretation of the results, these examinations must be repeated after an interval of at least 12 hours.

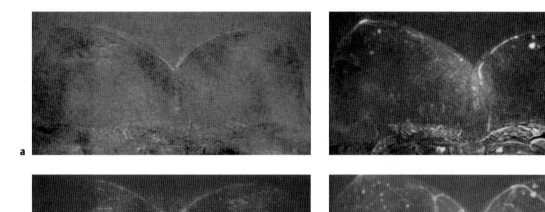

Fig. 6.2 a–d   Improper administration of contrast.
Paravenous administration of contrast (left) and repeat examination with correct contrast administration (right).
  a Subtraction images after improper administration of contrast.
  c MIP image. No pathological finding after paravasal contrast administration.

  b Correct contrast administration is documented by contrast in veins, in both internal mammary arteries, a small hypervascularized adenoma (left), and enhancement of the right nipple.
  d The contrasted veins are a definite indication of correct contrast administration.

Motion Artifacts

Motion artifacts seen in MR mammography have two major causes. One is the transmission of heart pulsations, which predominantly affects the left breast of slender patients. The other main cause is movement by the patient during the examination (Fig. 6.**3**). Breast compression using a special compression device (see Chapter 3, Figs. 3.**8**–3.**10**) reduces the degree of motion artifacts significantly (Fig. 6.**4**).

The quality of subtraction images is especially sensitive to motion artifacts during the dynamic measurements. The effect is generally seen as the presence of black and white ribbonlike zones lacking in image information. Such artifacts are occasionally seen in lesser degrees in the peripheral areas of the affected breast. They are also seen within the breast parenchyma, however, and more often near the pectoral muscle due to thoracic breathing movements.

When motion artifacts are present in the subtraction images, a careful inspection of the single images in their dynamic order is recommended. Evaluation of images with identical slice position in the so-called cine mode is useful for this purpose since motion artifacts are less disturbing when the corresponding images are viewed in rapid succession. If the presence of motion artifacts is extreme, the examination should be repeated at a later time.

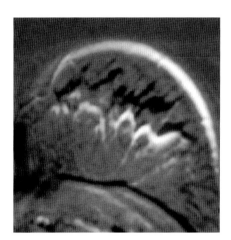

Fig. 6.**3** **Motion artifacts.**
Ribbonlike zones with signal loss (black) or signal summation (white) as a result of movement during the examination.

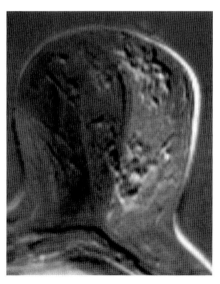

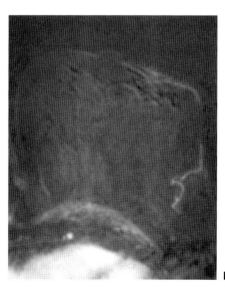

Fig. 6.**4 a, b** **Motion artifacts.**
a Artifacts oriented predominantly in the medio-lateral direction in an examination performed without a special compression device.
b Repeat examination with light compression using ventral padding. Elimination of motion artifacts.

a

b

Out-of-Phase Imaging

Protons bound in fat tissue possess a different resonance frequency from protons in water (or breast parenchyma). In MRI this produces an effect termed *chemical shift*. Especially in the GE sequences used in MR mammography, there results a phase difference between the signal of protons in water and that of protons in fat tissue. If this difference is 180°, it is referred to as out-of-phase imaging (or opposed-phase imaging). If the difference is 0°, then fat and water spins are in phase (in-phase imaging). The strength of this effect depends on the magnetic field strength.

Out-of-phase imaging results in signal loss at the borderlines between fat-containing and water-containing tissues. In dynamic MR imaging, this applies to the border between fat tissue and breast parenchyma. Depending upon the field strength of the system used, the echo time (TE) should be selected such that in-phase imaging results and interfering signal loss at these borders is avoided (Fig. 6.**5**).

Appropriate echo times for in-phase imaging dependent on magnetic field strength

Field strength 0.5 T: TE < 3.5 ms
Field strength 1.0 T: TE = 7.2 ms
Field strength 1.5 T: TE = 4.8 ms

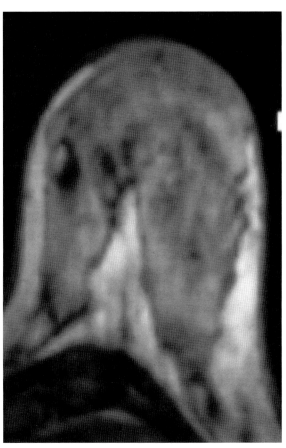 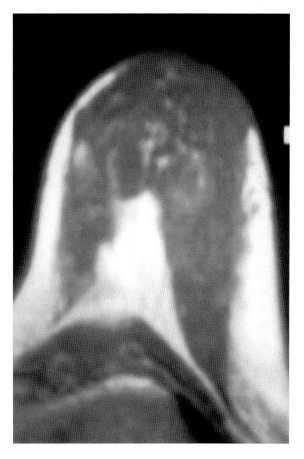

Fig. 6.**5 a, b   Artifacts caused by out-of-phase imaging.**
a Precontrast examination of the breast using a 1.5 T system. Signal loss artifacts at borderlines between fat and parenchyma due to inappropriate echo time (TE = 7.5 ms).

b Elimination of these artifacts by selection of correct echo time (TE = 5 ms).

Maladjustments of Transmitter and Receiver Settings

Maladjustment of the transmitter and receiver settings may lead to undesirable signal alterations of breast tissue during the repetitive measurements of a dynamic MR examination (Fig. 6.6). As a consequence, a signal increase, signal decrease, or fluctuations in signal intensity may occur and preclude a reasonable signal curve analysis during the postprocessing procedure. As a rule, therefore, no readjustment or tuning of the transmitter or receiver should be done between the performance of the precontrast examination and the taking of measurements after contrast administration. If such problems should arise, they can be recognized by the abnormal signal curve obtained by placing the ROI in an area of fat tissue, which shows no or little enhancement under physiological conditions.

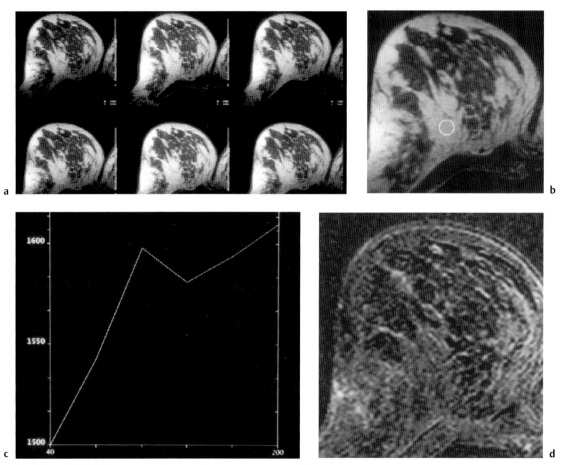

Fig. 6.**6 a–d   Maladjustments of transmitter and receiver settings.**
a Identical single slices in a dynamic examination with discrete fluctuations in the fat signal.
b Signal analysis in a ROI in fat tissue.
c Documentation of steady signal increase based on this analysis.
d Resulting subtraction image shows „negative image" with simulation of contrast enhancement within fat tissue and missing enhancement of parenchyma.

Susceptibility Artifacts

Susceptibility artifacts in the breast occur when ferro-magnetic foreign material lies within the breast or close to the thoracic wall. These artifacts are most commonly seen after use of an electrocauter during surgery (Fig. 6.**7**), which leaves fine metal abrasions in the tissue and causes typically round signal loss artifacts up to 10 mm in diameter in the MR image. The artifacts are so characteristic that previous surgery can be assumed even without access to the patient's history.

Other intramammary causes of susceptibility artifacts include broken needle parts after surgery, metal plates of prosthesis expanders, and metal clips used to mark the tumor bed after breast-conserving therapy. Extramammary causes include sternal wire cerclages after thoracic surgery (Fig. 6.**8**), belt buckles, and other metal objects on articles of clothing, which can result in extreme signal loss.

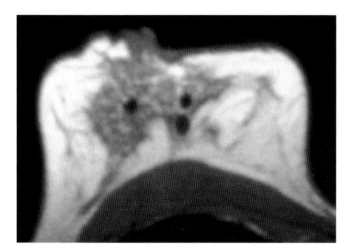

Fig. 6.**7** **Susceptibility artifacts.**
Perfectly round areas of signal loss after intraoperative hemostasis using an electrocauter.

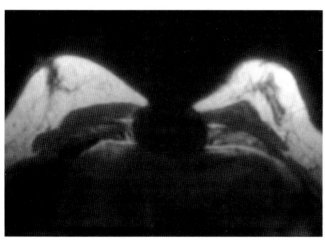

Fig. 6.**8** **Susceptibility artifact.**
Round signal loss due to sternal cerclage after thoracic surgery.

Cardiac Flow Artifacts

Cardiac flow artifacts are seen as an interfering, overlapping band of artifacts in the direction of the phase-encoding gradient. For the axial imaging plane, the phase-encoding gradient should be selected to be in the medio-lateral direction so that the cardiac artifact band crosses the image dorsally of the breasts through the thorax. Occasionally, however, parenchymal structures localized in the lateral areas of the breast and/or in the axillary tail may be incompletely imaged (i.e., obscured). This problem is sometimes encountered in patients with breast implants, which often reach far laterally, limiting the evaluation of the lateral areas of the implant and the surrounding parenchyma. In our experience it is advantageous in such cases to perform an additional measurement with a rotated phase-encoding gradient (in the ventro-dorsal direction) before the pre-contrast and after finishing the dynamic examination (Fig. 6.**9**). These two measurements can easily be differenced to provide a rough impression of the findings in the lateral areas of the prostheses and parenchyma despite the fact that the long time interval between the two measurements results in stronger motion artifacts. If an enhancing lesion is seen in this additional examination, a new appointment should be made to repeat the MR mammography examination with primary rotation of the phase-encoding gradient and performance of dynamic measurements.

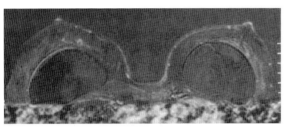
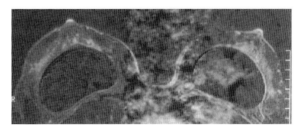

Fig. 6.**9 a, b   Cardiac flow artifacts.**
a Axial MR image with phase-encoding gradient in mediolateral direction. Limited evaluation of lateral breast and prosthesis areas due to cardiac motion artifacts (subtraction of precontrast image from second postcontrast image).

b Complete imaging of lateral breast and prosthesis areas in axial MR image with ventrodorsal rotation of phase-encoding gradient (subtraction of precontrast image from sixth postcontrast image). Acceptable level of motion artifacts.

Coil Artifacts

Dedicated breast coils available from most companies have the transmitting and receiving coils arranged in the form of circular elements that partially or completely surround the breasts in the coronary orientation. An increased signal occurs at the level of the coil windings, and the breast areas localized nearest to the coil show a higher signal intensity (Fig. 6.**10**). Normally, these effects are seen in the subcutaneous fat tissue and do not interfere with image interpretation. In breasts with an extremely high proportion of parenchyma to fat tissue and a thin subcutaneous layer of fat, misinterpretation of findings in the marginal parenchymal areas is possible. In cases with such questionable findings, these areas should be evaluated further using an adapted window setting.

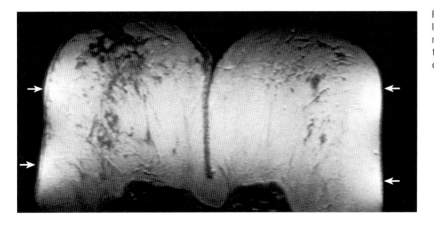

Fig. 6.**10   Coil artifacts.**
Increased signal intensity in the marginal areas of both breasts at the level of the circularly arranged coil windings (arrows).

Incorrect Region of Interest (ROI)

The semiquantitative evaluation of the signal changes after administration of contrast is performed in so-called regions of interest (ROIs). These measurement regions must be placed so that they include areas of maximal enhancement within a hypervascularized lesion and yet do not enclose less strongly enhancing areas, so as not to misrepresent the signal curve characteristics (Fig. 6.**11**). This is especially important for lesions with a ring-enhancement pattern. Here the ROI must be placed in the peripheral, strongly enhancing region of the lesion and not in the central, less vascularized necrotic or fibrotic areas. The recommended ROI size is between 2 and 5 pixels. In addition, it is sometimes necessary and prudent to perform several measurements using ROIs in differently enhancing areas within the same lesion. The signal curve with the most suspicious course should then be used for interpretation of the lesion.

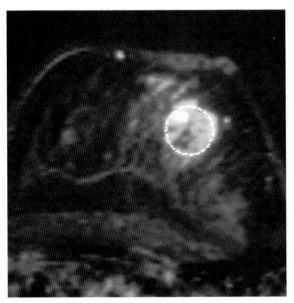

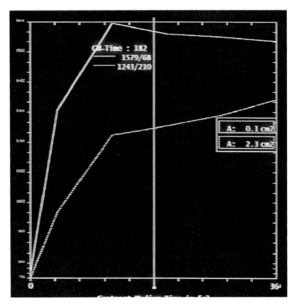

Fig. 6.**11 a,b   Placement of the ROI.**
Centrally localized, inhomogenous area of increased enhancement in the subtraction image of the left breast.
a Correct placement of a ROI within a maximally enhancing area of a hypervascularized lesion (small circle, area = 0.1 cm²), and placement of an unsuitable ROI (large circle, area = 2.3 cm²).

b The solid line with the steep initial increase and postinitial plateau represents the results from measurements using the correct ROI. The broken line illustrates the falsification of the signal curve characteristics if an unsuitable ROI including areas of weaker enhancement is selected.

Signal Alteration after Diagnostic Procedures

The performance of a diagnostic procedure on the breast may cause an alteration of the MR signal in both the precontrast image and the contrast-enhanced measurements. This may be an endotumoral or peritumoral signal increase in the T1-weighted measurement due to localized or diffuse hematomas (Fig. 6.**12**), or contrast enhancement as a result of hyperemia. Localized contrast enhancement may be segmental (e.g., after galactography) or diffuse (e.g., after several large-core biopsies or open biopsy) (Fig. 6.**13**). The medical history of the patient usually allows the correct interpretation of such changes.

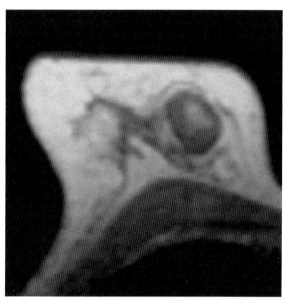

Fig. 6.**12   Endotumoral hematoma.**
Localized signal increase within a fibroadenoma after large-core biopsy. T1-weighted precontrast image.

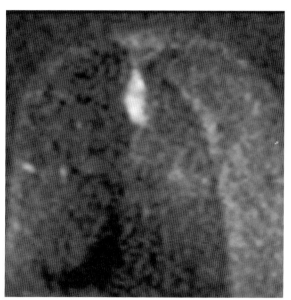

Fig. 6.**13   Segmental enhancement after galactography.**
Segmental enhancement increase three days after galactography. Image subtraction after contrast administration.

7 Normal Findings in MR Mammography

Morphology

The adult female breast is composed of three different tissue components: skin, subcutaneous tissue, and breast tissue (parenchyma and stroma). The skin is thin and contains hair follicles, sebaceous glands, and exocrine sweat glands. The *mammary papilla*, or *nipple*, contains sebaceous and exocrine sweat glands as well as abundant sensory nerve endings, but no hair follicles. The skin around the nipple constitutes the *areola* and is pigmented. Near its periphery are found elevations: *Morgagni's tubercles*, formed by the openings of the ducts of *Montgomery's glands*. These are large sebaceous glands that represent an intermediate type between sweat and mammary glands.

The parenchyma is divided into 15–20 cone-shaped lobes (*Lobi glandulae mammariae*), whose collecting ducts increase in diameter to form the subareolar lac- tiferous sinuses (*Ductus lactiferi colligentes*). Between 5 and 10 major collecting milk ducts open at the nipple. Each lobe is made up of 20–40 lobules (*Lobuli glandulae mammariae*) that consist of 10–100 alveoli or tubulosaccular secretory units.

The stroma of the breast contains varying amounts of fat, connective tissue, blood vessels, nerves, and lymphatics. *Stromal tissue* forms a mantel around the epithelial tissue of the lobes and along the peripheral ducts. Interlobular connective tissue surrounds the lobules and the central ducts. Fibrous bands called *Cooper's suspensory ligaments* connect the fascial tissue enveloping the breast with the deep pectoral fascia covering the pectoral major and anterior serratus muscles, and support the breast.

Blood Supply

Approximately 60% of the arterial blood supply to the breast, mostly to the medial quadrants and central portions, is provided by the perforating branches of the internal thoracic artery. Approximately 30% of arterial blood flow, chiefly to the upper outer quadrant, is supplied by the lateral mammary branches of the lateral thoracic artery (Fig. 7.1). Branches of the thora- coacromial, 3rd–5th intercostal, subscapular, and thoracodorsal arteries may also contribute to the arterial blood supply to a smaller extent. The fact that the blood supply to different areas of the breast derives from different arteries is of no importance in dynamic MR mammography.

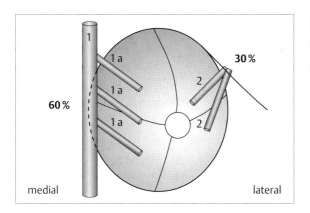

Fig. 7.**1 Arterial blood supply of the breast.**
The medial quadrants and central portions of the breast are supplied with arterial blood by the internal thoracic artery (1). The upper outer quadrant of the breast is supplied with arterial blood mainly by the lateral thoracic artery (2).

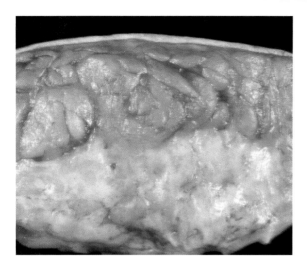

Fig. 7.**2**   **Comparison of macroanatomic dissection and MR mammographic image.**

a   Macroanatomic dissection of a normal breast.

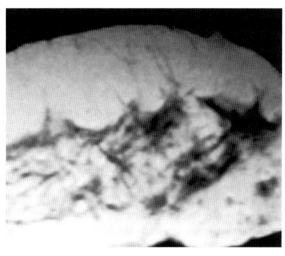

b   T1-weighted precontrast examination.

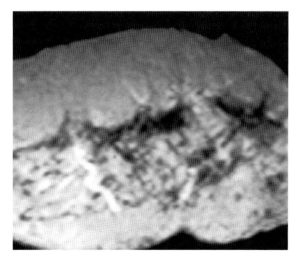

c   T2-weighted examination.

Parenchyma and Age

Morphological aspects of the female breast undergo fundamental changes that depend on age. The parenchymal changes occurring during pregnancy and the peripartal period will not be discussed here since they are not relevant for MR mammography.

Breast enlargement and development of the mammary ducts begins a few years before the menarche. Development of the lobuli, however, does not begin until one to two years after the menarche and continues through the 35th year of life. At this time the physiological process of breast involution with regressive lobular changes begins. Figures 7.3–7.6 show T1-weighted precontrast images as examples of the different developmental stages. It must be noted, however, that there is very great interindividual variability.

Contrast enhancement in MR mammography is significantly greater in women between the ages of 35 and 50 years compared to that in younger (<35 years) and older (>50 years) women. This is due to the greater incidence of adenomatous and fibrocystic breast changes found in women of this age group (Müller-Schimpfle et al. 1997).

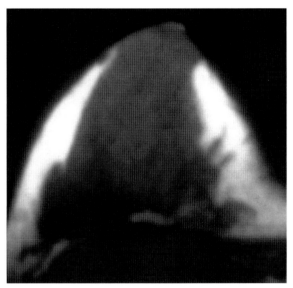

Fig. 7.3 **Juvenile breast (15 years). Dense parenchymal structures without fat inclusions.**

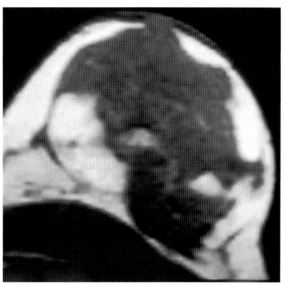

Fig. 7.4 **Breast of a mature woman (30 years) with dense parenchymal structures and singular fat inclusions.**

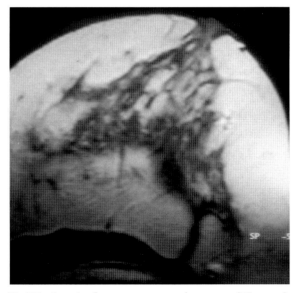

Fig. 7.5 **Breast of a premenopausal woman (50 years). Parenchyma is interspersed with fatty tissue.**

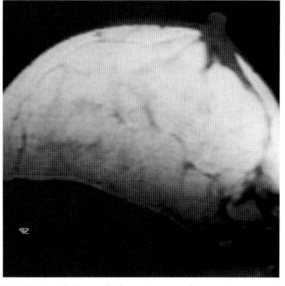

Fig. 7.6 **Involution of breast parenchyma in a postmenopausal woman (70 years).**

Parenchymal Asymmetry, Accessory Glandular Tissue

An *asymmetry* is defined as the presence of glandular tissue in an area of one breast without a corresponding parenchymal area in the contralateral breast (Fig. 7.**7**). Asymmetries are frequent findings in which one breast is often larger than the other (left > right more often than right > left). When no palpable mass is present and mammography shows no characteristic changes suggestive of malignancy, such an asymmetry is of no clinical significance.

Accessory glandular breast tissue does not have immediate contact with the main body of breast parenchyma.

Typically it is located in the axillary tail of one or both breasts and has a similar morphology to that of the remaining parenchyma (Fig. 7.**8**).

Parenchymal asymmetries and accessory glandular tissue normally show a slight CM uptake with a continuous increase over time in dynamic MR mammography, corresponding to the signal of normal breast parenchyma. If the course of the signal intensity curve demonstrates criteria suggestive of malignancy, then further evaluation is mandatory to rule out breast cancer with a diffuse infiltrating growth pattern.

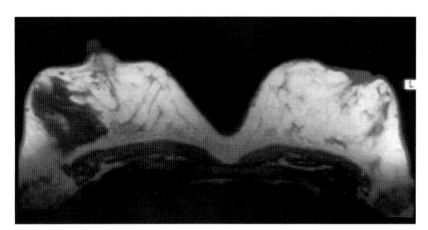

Fig. 7.**7** **Parenchymal asymmetry.**
Localized area of parenchyma in the right breast, complete involution of parenchyma in the left breast (precontrast T1-weighted GE sequence).

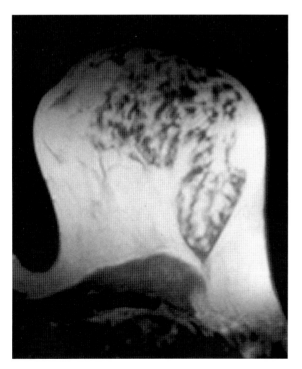

Fig. 7.**8** **Accessory glandular breast tissue.**
Additional parenchymal region in the axillary tail of the left breast, demonstrating identical internal structure to that of the remaining parenchyma (T1-weighted GE sequence, precontrast).

Nipple and Retromamillary Region

The nipple has a higher physiological CM uptake than the surrounding skin and breast parenchyma. This increased enhancement is typically found in the central portions of the nipple (Fig. 7.**9**) or linearly at the surface of the nipple (Fig. 7.**10**). The corresponding signal intensity curve usually shows a strong initial contrast enhancement (50–150% above precontrast level) and a continuous postinitial signal increase or plateau phase. The retromamillary region usually shows contrast enhancement equivalent to that of other normal parenchymal areas.

In contrast to the findings described above, increased enhancement of the entire nipple region, especially when a wash-out phenomenon is also present, represents a finding that must be correlated with the results of the clinical examination, ultrasound, and mammography in further evaluation (differential diagnosis: inflammation, Morbus Paget). Nodular enhancement areas with postinitial plateau or wash-out phenomenon in the retromamillary region are also abnormal findings and indicate the presence of a papilloma or other tumorous lesions.

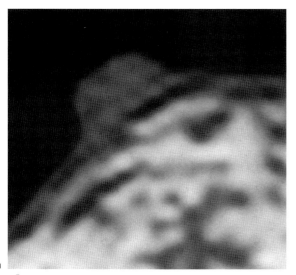

a

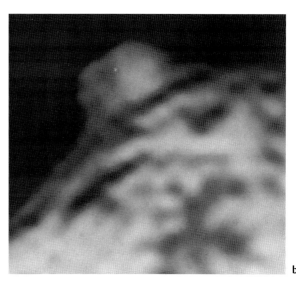

b

Fig. 7.**9 a, b Physiological contrast enhancement in the central portions of the nipple.**

a Precontrast T1-weighted examination.
b Image two minutes postcontrast.

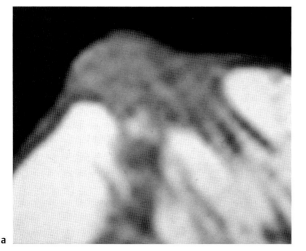

a

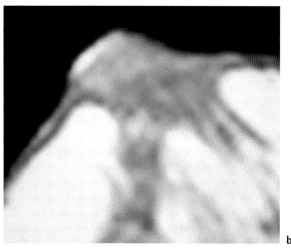

b

Fig. 7.**10 a, b Physiological contrast enhancement of the nipple, especially at the ventral surface.**

a Precontrast T1-weighted examination.
b Image two minutes postcontrast.

Interindividual Variations

There are strong interindividual differences in the level and distribution of CM uptake in the female breast and it is not possible to make a prospective estimation of the expected parenchymal enhancement after contrast administration. Neither palpation findings, parenchymal pattern in mammography, nor echogeneity in ultrasonography allows the selection of patients whose breast parenchyma will display an intense contrast enhancement pattern (Figs. 7.**11** and 7.**12**). Our own experience indicates that even examinations providing information about the vascularization (color-coded duplex sonography, contrast-enhanced color-coded duplex sonography) show no significant correlation with the parenchymal contrast enhancement pattern in MR mammography (Alamo et al. 1998).

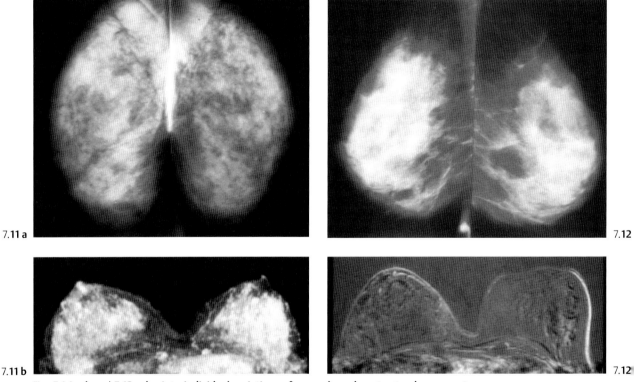

7.**11 a**

7.**12**

7.**11 b**

7.**12**

Figs 7.**1 1a, b** and 7.**12 a, b**   **Interindividual variations of parenchymal contrast enhancement.**
Comparison between two patients (Figs. 7.**11** and 7.**12**) with mammographically dense breast tissue (ACR [American College of Radiology] type 3 + 4).
a   Mammography.
b   Corresponding MR mammography shows extreme differences in CM uptake between these patients (subtraction images).

Intraindividual Fluctuations

Systematic longitudinal and cross-sectional studies show that parenchymal CM uptake is subject to intraindividual fluctuations (Fig. 7.**13**). In a comparative study in which MR mammography was performed once weekly within one menstrual cycle (20 healthy female volunteers, ages 21–35 years, average age 28 years), an enhancing lesion was demonstrated in 82 % of examined women. Of these lesions, 72 % were not seen in at least one of the four examinations (Kuhl et al. 1995). These results were supported by a study on a different group of patients (ages 27–55 years, average age 41.5 years) that compared CM uptake within the breast parenchyma (Müller-Schimpfle et al. 1997).

In consecutive MR mammography examinations performed at one-month intervals on another group of patients (ages 24–41 years, average age 34 years), 75 % of enhancing lesions were not demonstrated in at least one of the examinations performed (Kuhl et al. 1995). These studies reveal that, after contrast administration, signal intensity in the breast is subject to fluctuations from week to week as well as from month to month. The signal intensity curves of most of the enhancing lesions described in these studies showed typical characteristics of benign lesions, enabling the differentiation between benign and malignant lesions in the majority of cases.

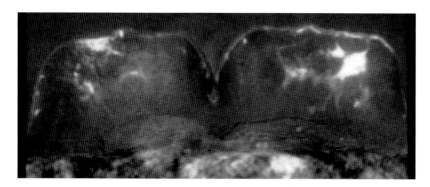

Fig. 7.**13 a, b   Intraindividual fluctuations of parenchymal contrast enhancement.**
Subtraction images.
a Pronounced increased focal enhancement, left > right. Third week of menstrual cycle.

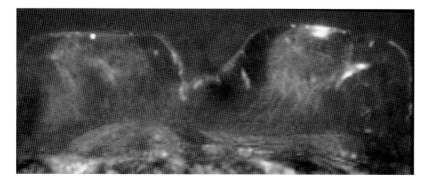

b Marked decrease of hypervascularized regions in repeat examination one month later (third week of menstrual cycle).

Hormone Replacement Therapy

Hormones influence the morphology, function, and vascularization of breast parenchyma. Hormone replacement therapy also affects the signal behavior in dynamic MR mammography (Fig. 7.**14**). Interindividual and intraindividual studies have shown that hormone replacement therapy in postmenopausal women results in increased parenchymal signal enhancement. It is significantly higher than that of women in the control group without hormone replacement therapy, and is comparable to that of premenopausal women.

Since there is no difference in the initial contrast enhancement of parenchyma in women with and without hormone replacement therapy, detection and differentiation of malignancy are not compromised. In women taking hormones, occasional problems have occurred in the differential diagnosis of focal enhancing lesions. Hormonal changes are reversible 4–8 weeks after discontinuing therapy, so that this interval should be observed when a repeat examination is planned to rule out malignancy. Further studies are needed to define the influence of different hormones on the signal behavior in MR mammography in more detail.

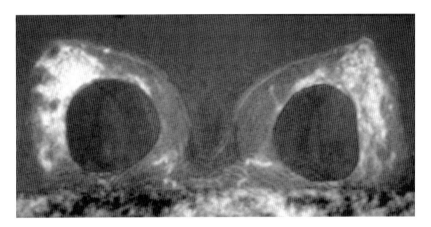

Fig. 7.**14 a, b Influence of hormone replacement therapy on contrast enhancement.**
a Strong enhancement of breast parenchyma in patient taking oral estrogens.

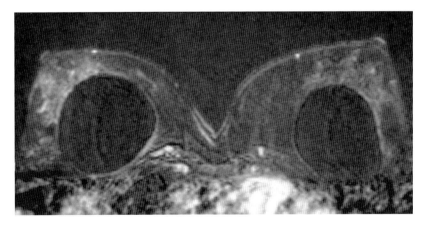

b Repeat examination three months after discontinuing hormone replacement therapy. Normalization of parenchymal CM uptake. Note bilateral silicone implants.

Pregnancy and the Lactating Breast

During pregnancy and the following lactation period, the female breast is subject to strong hormonal stimulation. As a result, the parenchyma of the breast shows a pronounced CM uptake in dynamic MR mammography. This has been demonstrated in the results of the few examinations performed on nursing women (Fig. 7.**15**). The use of MR mammography for examining pregnant women is additionally limited by the necessity of administering paramagnetic CM. For these reasons, the diagnostic work-up of ambiguous lesions during pregnancy and the nursing period should employ other diagnostic methods. It is advisable to avoid performing MR mammography in these phases.

MR mammography should also be avoided when early pregnancy cannot be ruled out. The diagnostic indications for MR mammography are never acutely life-threatening, so when pregnancy is a possibility either a pregnancy test must be performed or the examination should be delayed for a few weeks.

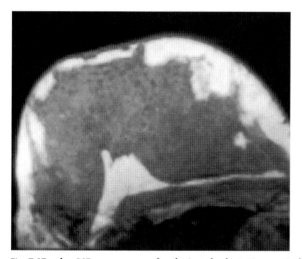 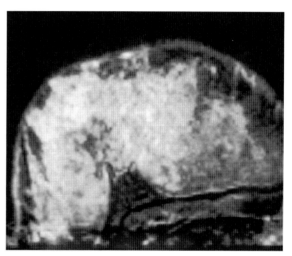

Fig. 7.**15 a, b   MR mammography during the lactation period.**
a Pronounced parenchyma without suspicious findings in the precontrast examination (T1-weighted FLASH sequence).

b Subtraction image showing extremely intense contrast enhancement of entire parenchymal body.

8 Benign Changes

Papillomas

Papillomas are characterized histopathologically as intraductal tumors composed of benign epithelial cells covering a central branching fibrovascular core. They are generally differentiated to include **solitary intraductal papillomas** (Figs. 8.**1**, 8.**2**, 8.**4**, and 8.**5**), which are located in the retromamillary region, and the small **peripheral intraductal papillomas**, which are usually multiple in number (Fig. 8.**3**).

Pseudopapillary lesions, which are intraductal hyperplasias with a papillary architecture that occur without the presence of a central fibrous core, and the **papillary adenoma of the nipple**, with its combination of papillary and tubular structures, should be distinguished from thesepapillomas . The pseudopapillary lesions include **papillomatosis** and **juvenile papillomatosis**, which commonly occurs in adolescents and young women between 10 and 40 years of age.

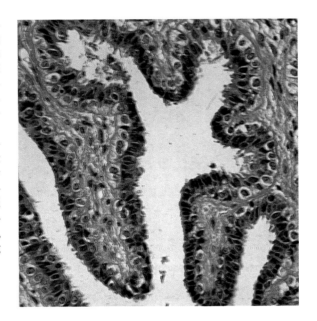

General information

Incidence:	Rare, 1–2% of all benign tumors.
Age peak:	4th–5th decade of life.
Risk of malignant transformation:	Not increased for solitary intraductal papillomas + papillary adenoma of the nipple; approx. 8% in 10 years for peripheral intraductal papillomas.

Findings

Clinical:	Spontaneous or provokable nipple discharge (exfoliative cytology). Rare occurrence of palpable mass (e.g., „ large retromammillary papillomas).
Mammography:	Usually occult lesion. Rarely well-circumscribed mass.
Galactography (method of choice):	Intraductal contrast exclusion(s) or abrupt duct ending(s).
Ultrasonography:	Usually occult lesion. Rarely round lesion in retromamillary region.

Clinical significance

Although papillomas represent benign lesions, imaging techniques cannot reliably rule out malignancy. Histological examination is therefore advisable.

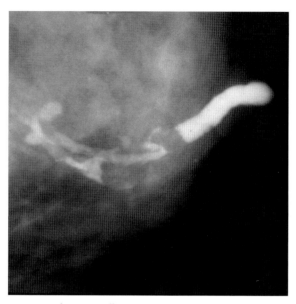

Fig 8.**1** **Solitary papilloma.**
Galactography showing intraductal contrast exclusion in retromamillary duct.

 MR mammography: Papilloma(s)

T1-weighted sequence (precontrast)
Small solitary intraductal papilloma:
Usually not detectable in precontrast image.

Larger solitary intraductal papilloma (> 1 cm):
Round or oval lesion with signal isointense to parenchyma.

Peripheral intraductal papillomas:
Usually not detectable in precontrast image.

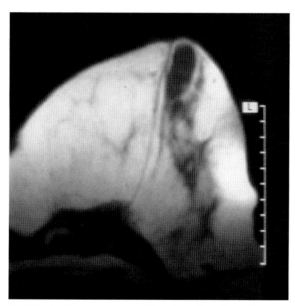 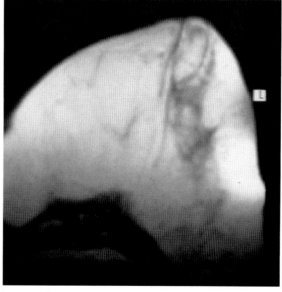

Fig. 8.**2a, b** **Large retromamillary intraductal papilloma.**
a Oval lesion of size ~2 × 3 cm in T1-weighted sequence. Signal isointense with parenchyma.

b Second measurement after contrast administration shows strong inhomogeneous signal enhancement within the lesion. Note that parenchyma also shows contrast enhancement.
Histology: Solitary intraductal papilloma.

MR mammography: Papilloma(s)

T1-weighted sequence (contrast-enhanced)
Round or oval lesion with homogeneous or inhomogeneous contrast enhancement, depending on
the size of the papilloma. Well-circumscribed.
Stronger initial contrast enhancement than surrounding parenchyma in most cases. Continuous
postinitial signal increase during entire examination period, occasionally postinitial plateau. Normally no wash-out phenomenon.

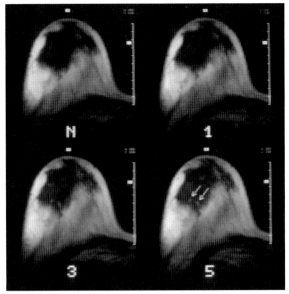

Fig. 8.**3** **Peripheral intraductal papillomas.**
The dynamic examination shows continuous contrast enhancement in two small lesions in the central portion of the right
breast (arrows).
Histology (surgery performed because of carcinoma at another
location): Intraductal papillomas.

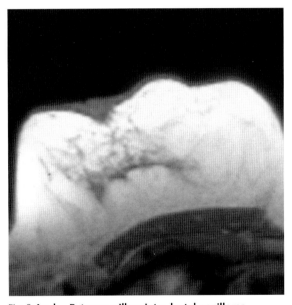

Fig. 8.**4 a, b** **Retromamillary intraductal papilloma.**
a No detection of isointense lesion in T1-weighted precontrast examination.

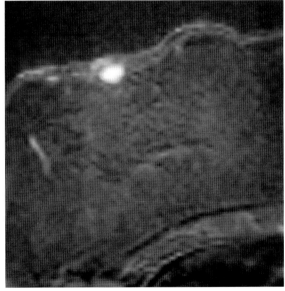

b Documentation of oval, well-circumscribed lesion in retromamillary region in subtraction image after contrast administration.
Histology: Intraductal papilloma.

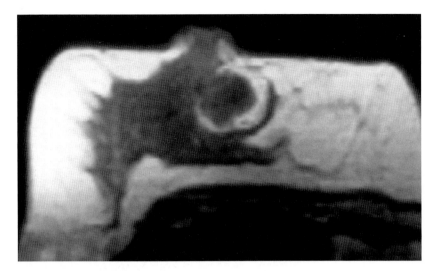

Fig. 8.**5a–d   Intraductal papilloma.**

a   Well-circumscribed lesion within cystic structure containing signal intense fluid in T1-weighted precontrast image.

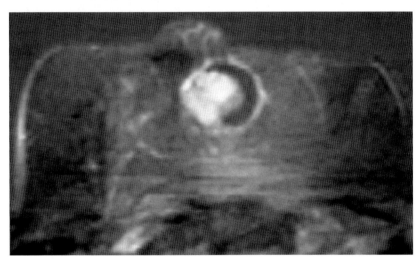

b   Subtraction image after contrast administration shows inhomogeneous enhancement in lesion and cyst wall.

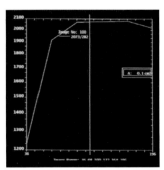

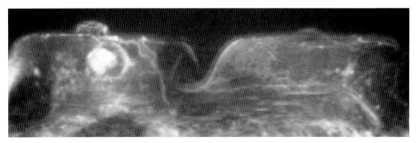

d   MIP image.
Histology: 2.5 cm intraductal papilloma in hemorrhagic cyst.

c   Signal analysis reveals an initial increase of 70 % with postinitial plateau.

Adenomas

Adenomas of the breast (Figs. 8.**6** and 8.**7**) are composed of benign epithelial elements with a sparse stromal component, features that differentiate them from fibroadenomas. Adenomas are commonly divided into two major groups: **tubular adenomas** and **lactating adenomas**. *Tubular adenomas* present in young women as well-circumscribed tumors and are composed of a proliferation of small tubular structures separated from adjacent breast tissue by an enveloping pseudocapsule. *Lactating adenomas* develop during pregnancy or the postpartum period and are composed of glands with secretory activity.

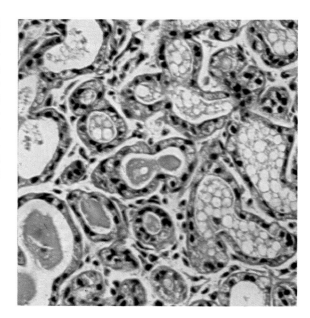

General information

Incidence:	Very rare benign breast tumor.
Age peak:	Especially younger women.
Risk of malignant transformation:	No proven data.
Multifocality:	Very rare.

Findings

Clinical:	Well-circumscribed, movable, painless mass.
Mammography:	Well-circumscribed, homogeneously dense lesion (round, oval, or lobulated), possible halo sign.
	Occasional macrocalcifications, less likely than in fibroadenomas.
Ultrasonography:	Well-circumscribed, oval lesion with homogeneous internal echo texture.
	Moderate to strong posterior acoustic enhancement, possible bilateral acoustic shadowing.
	No or slight lesion compressibility.

Clinical significance

Adenomas of the breast show similar characteristics to fibroadenomas in the various imaging techniques. If there is uncertainty about the histology, further diagnostic procedures are indicated to rule out malignancy (e.g., percutaneous biopsy).

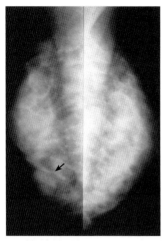

Fig. 8.**6** **Adenoma.** Mammographically dense parenchyma. Well-circumscribed, oval, homogeneous lesion near the skin in the right breast (arrow).

 MR mammography: Adenoma

T1-weighted sequence (precontrast)
Well-circumscribed, rounded lesion with isointense or slightly hypointense signal in comparison to breast parenchyma.

T2-weighted sequence
Strong signal intensity in most cases (comparable to the signal intensity of myxoid fibroadenomas).

T1-weighted sequence (contrast-enhanced)
Round or oval shape. Well-circumscribed borders. Usually homogeneous contrast enhancement. No ring enhancement. In most cases strong initial contrast enhancement (sometimes several hundred percent) with continuous postinitial signal increase or plateau.

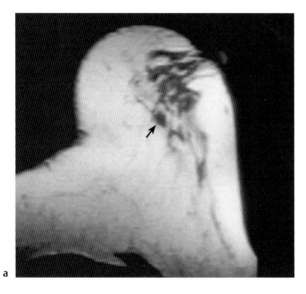

a

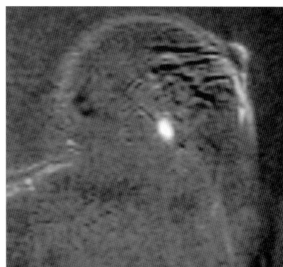

b

Fig. 8.**7a–c** **Adenoma.**
a Oval lesion with hypointense signal in precontrast T1-weighted image (arrow).
b Homogeneous CM uptake, well-circumscribed borders.
c Moderate initial contrast enhancement with continuous postinitial increase.
Histology: Tubular adenoma of the breast.

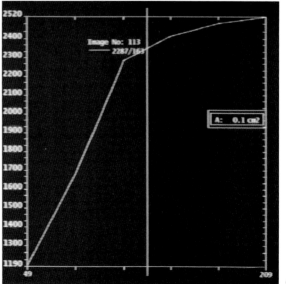

c

Fibroadenoma

Fibroadenomas (Fig. 8.**8**) are mixed fibroepithelial tumors. Depending on the endotumoral distribution of the stromal and epithelial components, they are classified as **intracanalicular** and **pericanalicular fibroadenomas**. This differentiation is of no clinical importance. In younger women, fibroadenomas typically have a high proportion of epithelial tissue. With increasing age, and especially in postmenopausal women, the fibrotic component of these tumors predominates and may exhibit progressive hyalinization and calcification (Figs. 8.**14**–**15**, and 8.**18**).

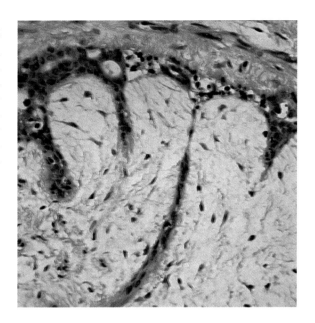

General information

Incidence:	Most common benign breast tumor (~10 % of all women).
Age peak:	All ages, peak between 20 and 50 years.
Risk of malignant transformation:	Very low (factor 1.3–1.9).
Multifocality:	10–15 %.

Findings

Clinical:	Well-circumscribed, movable, painless mass.
Mammography:	Well-circumscribed, homogeneously dense lesion (round, oval, or lobulated), possible halo sign.
	Endotumoral popcorn macrocalcifications (>2 mm).
	Cave: Endotumoral or peritumoral pleomorphic microcalcifications (differential diagnosis: carcinoma).
Ultrasonography:	Well-circumscribed, oval lesion with homogeneous internal echo texture.
	Moderate to strong posterior acoustic enhancement, possible bilateral acoustic shadowing.
	Macrocalcifications may cause complete posterior acoustic extinction.
	Compressibility of lesion: slight to good, depending on histological composition.

Clinical significance

Fibroadenomas must be differentiated from well-defined malignant tumors, especially in older women. If there is uncertainty about the histology, further diagnostic procedures are indicated to rule out malignancy (e.g., percutaneous biopsy).

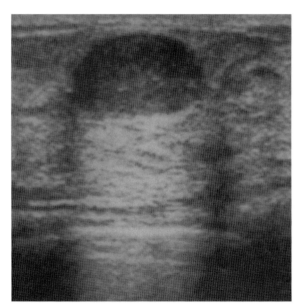

Fig. 8.**8**   **Fibroadenoma.**
Ultrasound shows well-circumscribed, oval lesion with homogeneous internal echo texture and narrow bilateral posterior shadowing.

 MR mammography: Fibroadenoma

T1-weighted sequence (precontrast)
Well-circumscribed round, oval, or lobulated lesion. Isointense or slightly hypointense signal in comparison to breast parenchyma. If located within parenchymal body, therefore, it is difficult or impossible to detect (Fig. 8.**9**). If located within fatty tissue, lesion appears more obvious (Fig. 8.**10**). In rare cases, endotumoral signal loss due to macrocalcifications (Fig. 5.**1c**).

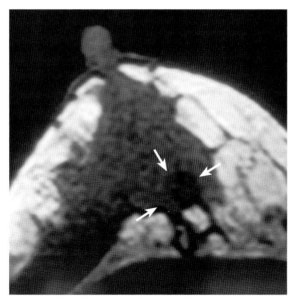

Fig. 8.**9**   **Fibroadenoma within parenchyma.**
Difficult detection of fibroadenoma due to only slightly lower signal intensity of lesion (arrows) compared to surrounding parenchyma in T1-weighted precontrast image.

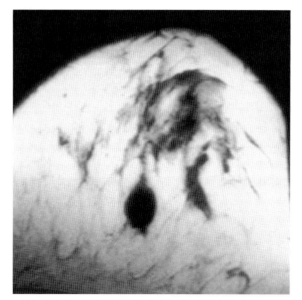

Fig. 8.**10**   **Fibroadenoma within fatty tissue.**
Clear demarcation of oval fibroadenoma within surrounding signal-intense fatty tissue in T1-weighted precontrast image.

MR mammography: Fibroadenoma

T2-weighted sequence

Signal behavior is dependent upon the histological composition of the fibroadenoma:

When a high proportion of epithelial tissue is present (more often in younger women), signal intensity is often high, making the differentiation from a cyst difficult (Fig. 8.**11**). Occasionally endo-tumoral septations, correlating to fibrotic tumor components, are seen (**Note**: The selection of a wide window is important!).

When a high proportion of the tumor is fibrotic (more often seen in older women), the fibroadenoma is usually not detectable because of the isointensity or slight hypointensity of the signal in comparison to the surrounding parenchyma (Fig. 8.**12**).

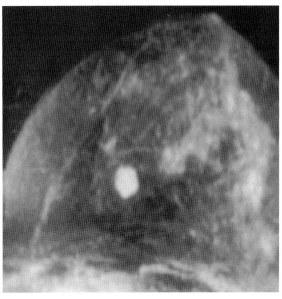 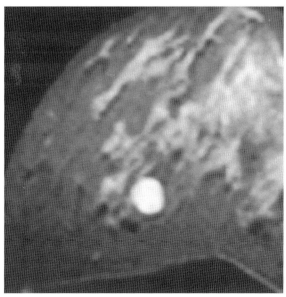

Fig. 8.**11 a, b Fibroadenoma with high epithelial component.**
a Subtraction image demonstrating hypervascularized lesion.

b T2-weighted image showing high signal intensity of lesion.
Histology: Myxoid fibroadenoma.

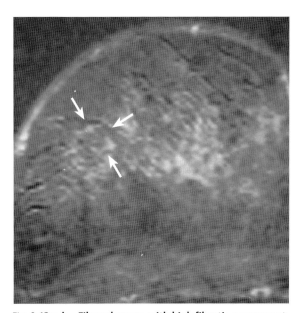 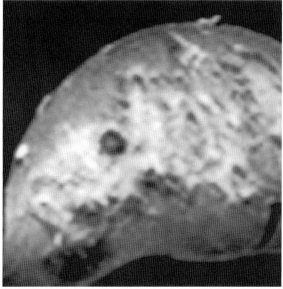

Fig. 8.**12 a, b Fibroadenoma with high fibrotic component.**
a Subtraction image demonstrating hypovascularized lesion (arrows).

b T2-weighted image showing predominantly hypointense lesion.
Unchanged over several years in ultrasonography.

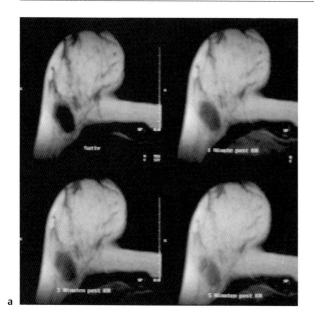

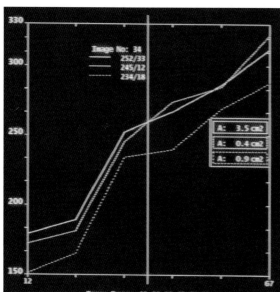

Fig. 8.**13 a, b   Hypovascularized fibroadenoma.**
a   Oval lesion within fatty tissue in the upper outer quadrant of
the right breast. Very slow CM uptake within the lesion
during dynamic examination. Dynamic images before and 1,
3, and 5 minutes after CM administration.
b   The signal curve analysis shows slight initial contrast enhancement (<50%) and continuous postinitial signal increase (in several ROIs).
Histology: Fibroadenoma.

 MR mammography: Fibroadenoma

T1-weighted sequence (contrast-nhanced)
The signal behavior of a fibroadenoma after contrast administration is dependent upon the histological composition of the tumor:

Tumors with a high proportion of epithelial tissue
(more frequent in younger women) show pronounced contrast enhancement. The strong initial
contrast enhancement (up to several hundred
percent of precontrast value) occasionally reaches
values higher than those found in many malignant
tumors. The postinitial signal usually displays a
continuous increase or plateau. A wash-out phenomenon is extremely rare (<1% in our collective). Endotumoral septations with slight CM uptake represent linearly distributed fibrotic tumor
portions (see Fig. 8.**17**). In rare cases, a nonenhancing peripheral border is seen as the expression of a pseudocapsular demarcation (MR equivalent of halo sign) (see Fig. 8.**16**).

Tumors with high proportion of fibrotic tissue
(more often in older women) (Fig. 8.**13**) show
no or slight CM uptake. There is correspondingly
no or slight contrast enhancement after contrast
administration with no or continuous postinitial
signal increase during the examination. Differentiation from carcinoma is usually unproblematic.

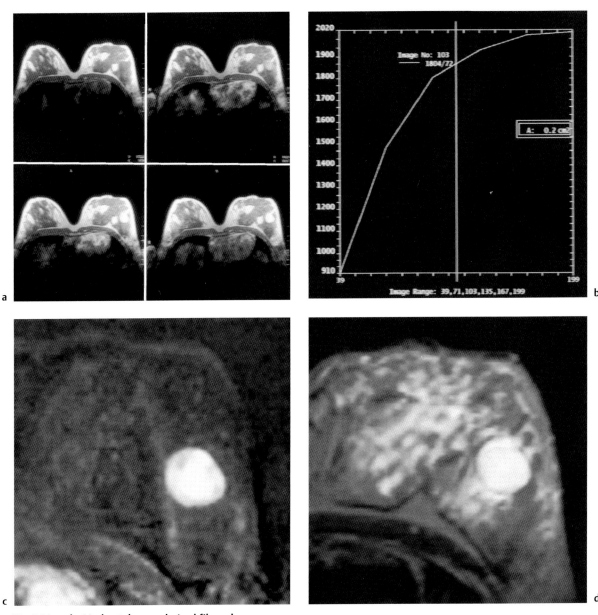

Fig. 8.**14 a– d Moderately vascularized fibroadenoma.**
Lesion located in upper outer quadrant of left breast.
a Documentation of lesion with continuous contrast enhancement after CM administration. Dynamic images before and 1, 3, and 5 minutes after CM administration.
b Initial contrast enhancement just under 100 % with continuous postinitial signal increase.

c Subtraction image shows round, well-circumscribed lesion with inhomogeneous contrast enhancement.
d T2-weighted image demonstrates lesion with strong signal. Histology: Fibroadenoma.

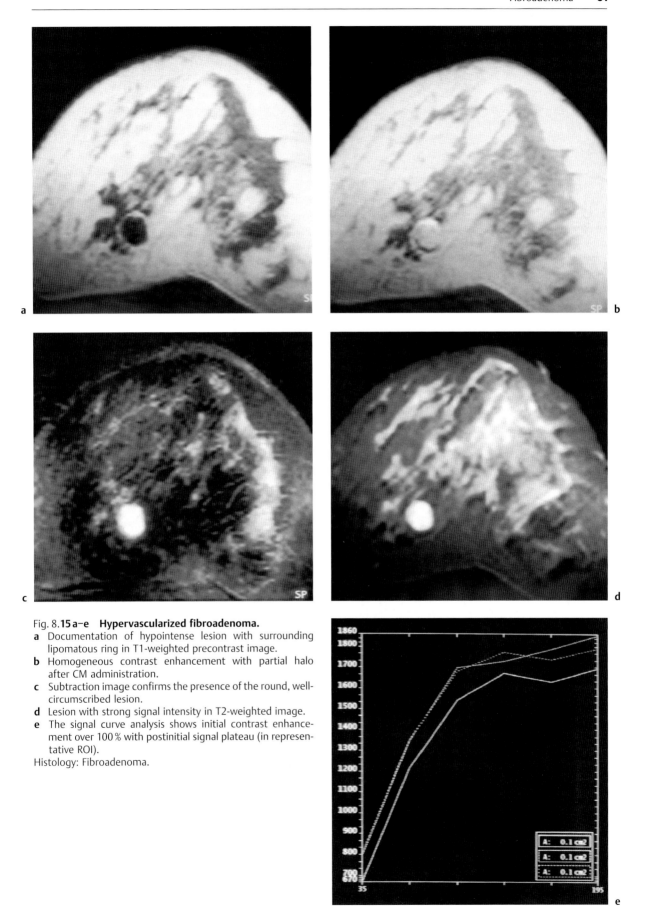

Fig. 8.15 a–e   Hypervascularized fibroadenoma.
a Documentation of hypointense lesion with surrounding lipomatous ring in T1-weighted precontrast image.
b Homogeneous contrast enhancement with partial halo after CM administration.
c Subtraction image confirms the presence of the round, well-circumscribed lesion.
d Lesion with strong signal intensity in T2-weighted image.
e The signal curve analysis shows initial contrast enhancement over 100 % with postinitial signal plateau (in representative ROI).
Histology: Fibroadenoma.

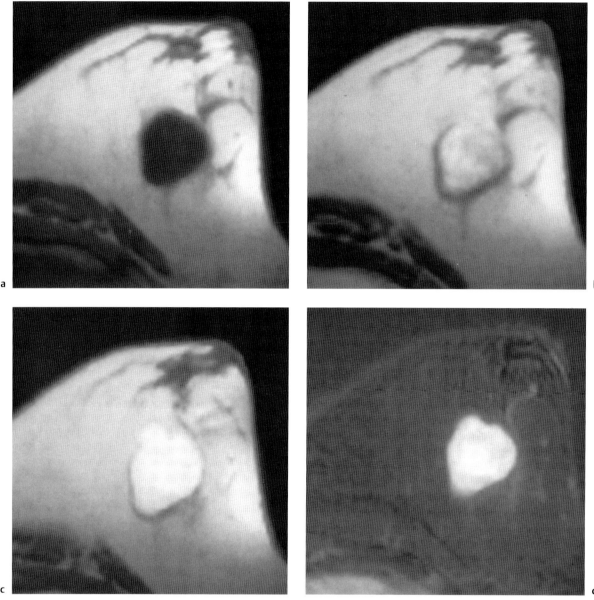

Fig. 8.**16 a–d   Hypervascularized fibroadenoma with halo sign.**
a T1-weighted precontrast image shows oval lesion with low signal intensity within adipose tissue.
b Two minutes after CM administration. Lesion demonstrates inhomogeneous CM uptake and semicircular border (partial halo) without contrast enhancement.
c Five minutes after CM administration. Continuous signal increase within lesion, persisting nonenhancing border.
d Documentation of lesion in subtraction image (second postcontrast measurement minus precontrast measurement).
Histological correlate of signal-free border: Streaks of fibrosis in marginal areas of a fibroadenoma.

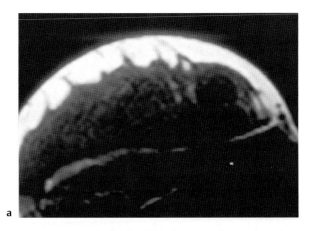
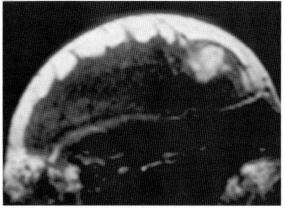

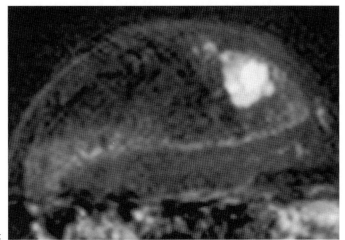
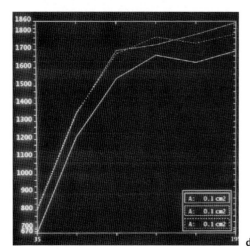

Fig. 8.**17 a–d   Fibroadenoma with endotumoral septations.**

a T1-weighted precontrast image shows discrete rounded lesion with hypointense signal in comparison with surrounding parenchyma.

b The first measurement after CM administration shows pronounced enhancement within lesion, now appearing lobulated, and demarcation of less vascularized septations.

c Subtraction image confirms lobulated lesion and endotumoral septations.

d Signal curve analysis using several representative ROIs shows strong initial contrast enhancement over 100% with continuous postinitial signal increase i.e. plateau.

Histology: Fibroadenoma.

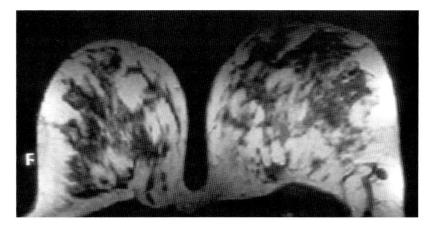

Fig. 8.**18 a–d   Small hypervascularized fibroadenoma.**
a   T1-weighted image with documentation of round hypointense lesion within adipose tissue in outer portion of left breast.

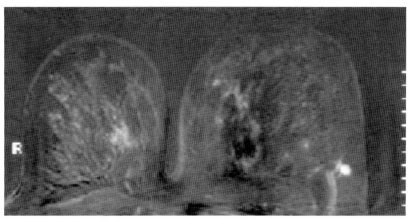

b   Homogeneous contrast enhancement within lesion after CM administration.

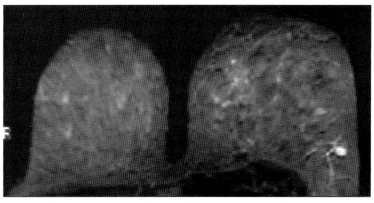

c   T2-weighted image showing lesion with hyperintense signal.

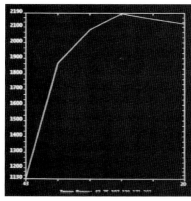

d   Signal curve analysis shows moderate initial contrast enhancement with postinitial plateau.
Histology: Fibroadenoma.

Variants of Fibroadenomas

The following variants exist in addition to the common adult type of fibroadenoma:

Juvenile fibroadenomas are Rapidly growing lesions that appear during adolescence, i.e., puberty (Fig. 8.**19**). They make up ~0.5% to 2% of all fibroadenomas.

Giant fibroadenomas are large lesions with a diameter >5 cm. They appear with a higher frequency during pregnancy and the lactating period.

 MR mammography: Variants of fibroadenomas

T1-weighted sequence (precontrast)
Round, oval, or lobulated lesion with isointense or slightly hypointense signal in comparison with parenchyma.

T2-weighted sequence
Typically hyperintense signal behavior.

T1-weighted sequence (contrast-enhanced)
Strong contrast enhancement, comparable to fibroadenomas with a high proportion of epithelial tissue. Sharp demarcation from surrounding tissue.

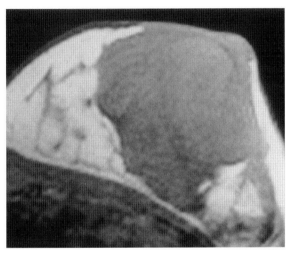
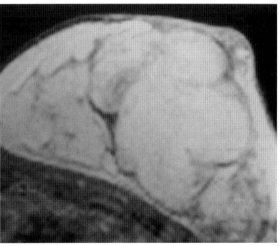

Fig. 8.19 a, b   Juvenile (giant) fibroadenoma.
a T1-weighted precontrast image allows no differentiation between a solid tumor and normal breast parenchyma.

b Pronounced contrast enhancement in well-circumscribed tumor with endotumoral septations (second measurement after CM administration). Surgical indication for cosmetic reasons.
Histology: Fibroadenoma.

Benign Phyllodes Tumor

(Synonyms: benign phylloides tumor, fibroadenoma phyllodes)

The phyllodes tumor is a distinctive fibroepithelial tumor of the breast without counterpart in any other organ of the body (Figs. 8.**20** and 8.**21**). The benign form of this tumor is characterized by its structural similarity to the fibroadenoma, a low mitotic activity (0–4 mitoses/10 fields of view at 400× magnification [high-power field; HPF]), no nuclear atypia, and a tumor growth pattern that displaces the surrounding tissue. The stroma of the tumor can show fibrous, lipoid, myxoid, and muscular differentiation. In addition, the tumor often shows signs of hemorrhage and ulceration.

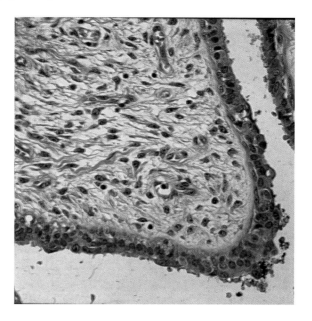

General information

Incidence:	0.3% of all breast tumors.
Age peak:	30–50 years
Risk of malignant transformation:	No increased risk. **Note**: High local recurrence rate of ~30%.

Findings

Clinical:	Rapidly growing, smooth or tuberous mass, up to 10 cm or more in diameter. Skin changes with large tumors (thinning and/or livid discoloration).
Mammography:	Homogeneous, round, oval, or lobulated tumor (similar to fibroadenoma). Occasional halo sign due to compression of surrounding tissue. Rarely microcalcifications or macrocalcifications.
Ultrasonography:	Well-circumscribed, rounded, or lobulated lesion with posterior acoustic enhancement. Cystic inclusions diagnostically relevant.

Clinical significance

The differential diagnosis between a phyllodes tumor and a fibroadenoma is occasionally difficult. Rapid growth and the documentation of cystic inclusions are indicative for a phyllodes tumor.

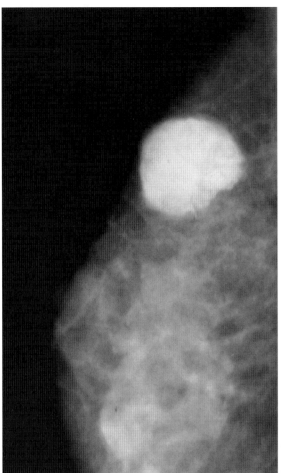

 MR mammography: Benign phyllodes tumor

T1-weighted sequence (precontrast)

Well-circumscribed lesion without pseudocapsular demarcation. Signal intensity equivalent to that of parenchyma. Occasional documentation of rounded inclusions with comparatively hypointense signal as MR equivalent of cystic or necrotic changes.

T2-weighted sequence

Well-circumscribed lesion with isointense to hyperintense signal in comparison to parenchymal signal intensity. Occasional documentation of rounded inclusions with hyperintense signal as MR equivalent of cystic or necrotic changes.

T1-weighted sequence (contrast-enhanced)

Strong contrast enhancement within solid tumor portions. Increasing demarcation of existing cystic or necrotic areas in the further course of the examination. Initial contrast enhancement is usually 100% or more. The postinitial signal usually shows a continuous increase or plateau. When no liquid inclusions are documented, differentiation from a fibroadenoma with a high proportion of epithelial tissue is not possible. Differentiation of this benign lesion from a *malignant phyllodes tumor* or a *borderline phyllodes tumor* is not possible in MR mammography.

◁ Fig. 8.**20 Benign phyllodes tumor.**
Mammography shows large, well-circumscribed, lobulated mass with homogeneous high density.

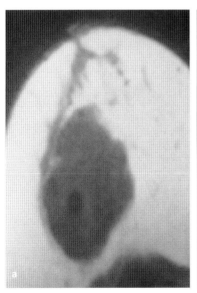 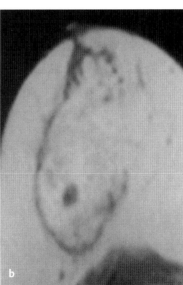 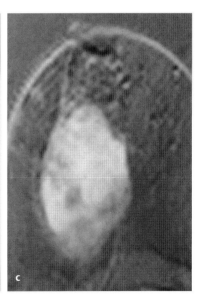

Fig. 8.**21 a–c Benign phyllodes tumor.**

a T1-weighted precontrast image shows oval, well-circumscribed lesion within surrounding adipose tissue.

b Strong contrast enhancement with demarcation of nonenhancing cystic inclusion after CM administration. No contrast enhancement in portions of the tumor border.

c Documentation of lesion in subtraction image.
Histology: Benign phyllodes tumor of the right breast.

Lipomas

Lipomas of the breast are compossed of encapsulated nodules containing mature fat cells (Figs. 8.**22** and 8.**23**). These rare lesions must be differentiated from mixed tumors with macroscopically visible adipose tissue.

Intramammary lipomas can be differentiated from lipomas of extramammary location (Fig. 8.**24**).

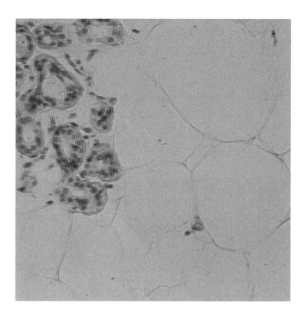

___ **General information**

Incidence:	Extremely rare.
Age peak:	All ages.
Risk of malignant transformation:	No increased risk.

___ **Findings**

Clinical:	Often occult.
	Occasionally soft, more rarely firm, movable mass.
Mammography (method of choice):	Well-circumscribed, fully or partially encapsulated radiolucent tumor.
Ultrasonography:	Hypoechoic or hyperechoic lesion seen only when of large size.

___ **Clinical significance**

Lipomas of the breast are very rare, usually clinically occult lesions, often demonstrated solely in mammography as a side finding. The mammographic appearance is pathognomonic. Further diagnostic examinations are therefore not necessary.

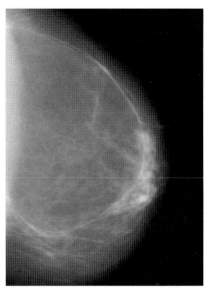

T1-weighted sequence (precontrast)
Well-circumscribed lesion with hyperintense signal (fat-equivalent). Possible documentation of thin, hypointense capsule. No nonadipose internal structures.

T2-weighted sequence
Well-circumscribed lesion with signal intensity equivalent to that of subcutaneous fat.

T1-weighted sequence (contrast-enhanced)
No contrast enhancement.

Fig. 8.**22 Lipoma of the breast.**
Mammography shows well-circumscribed, encapsulated lesion with radiolucent density. Displacement of surrounding parenchymal structures.

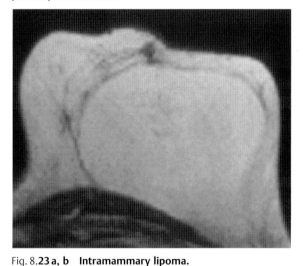

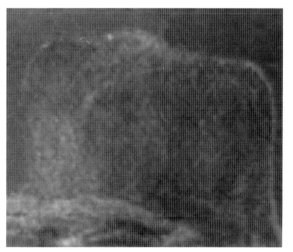

Fig. 8.**23 a, b   Intramammary lipoma.**
a T1-weighted precontrast image showing large lesion with fat-equivalent signal and encompassing hypointense capsule.

b Subtraction image demonstrates absence of contrast enhancement.
No histological examination.

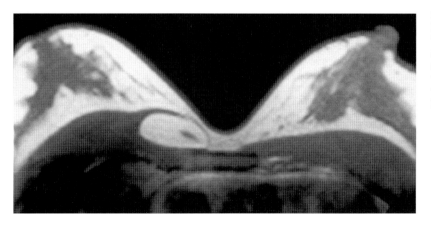

Fig. 8.**24   Extramammary lipoma.**
T1-weighted precontrast sequence showing spindle-shaped, well-circumscribed tumor with fat-equivalent signal within the pectoral muscle group.
No histological examination.

Fibrocystic Breast Tissue

Fibrocystic changes of the breast, previously referred to as *mammary dysplasia*, describe the proliferation of hormone-dependent mesenchymal and epithelial structures in the mammary gland. Fibrocystic changes encompass a heterogeneous group of abnormalities that may occur separately or together. The morphological components, present in various degrees, comprise cysts, lobular hyperplasia, adenosis, ductal and alveolar hyperplasia (papillomatosis or epitheliosis), and stromal fibrosis (Fig. 8.**25**). The etiology of such changes is presumed to be a hormonal imbalance. Fibrocystic breast tissue is classified into three groups by Dupont and Page (Table 8.**1**).

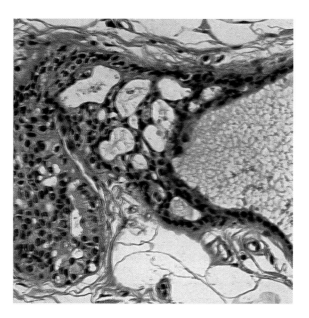

Table 8.**1**   Classification of Fibrocystic Breast Changes into Three Groups (Dupont and Page[1])

Grade	Histological Category	Risk of Breast Cancer
I (~70%)	Nonproliferative lesions	Not increased
II (~25%)	Proliferative lesions without atypia	Increased by a factor of 2
III (~5%)	Proliferative lesions with atypia	Increased by a factor of 4–5

[1] Dupont and Page 1985; Page et al. 1985.

___

— **General information**

Incidence: ~50% of all women.
Age peak: 40–60 years.

— **Findings**

Clinical:	Variable (from none to palpable masses of different sizes and increased diffuse breast firmness). Symmetrical findings in most cases. Fluctuation with the menstrual cycle.
Mammography:	Often diffuse, rarely circumscribed structural hyperdensities. Symmetrical findings in most cases. Macrocalcifications and microcalcifications (differentiation between benign and malignant lesions sometimes difficult).
Ultrasonography:	Increased hyperechoic structures. Multiple hypoechoic tubular patterns (dilated ductal structures), often multiple anechoic lesions with posterior/distal acoustic enhancement (cysts), Symmetrical findings in most cases.

— **Clinical significance**

Imaging techniques do not allow reliable differentiation between the different types of fibrocystic changes. It is therefore not possible to make an accurate assessment of a woman's risk of breast cancer by these methods.

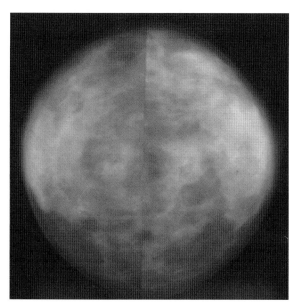

Fig. 8.**25 Fibrocystic changes.**
Mammogram shows extremely dense breast tissue in woman with proliferative changes.

 MR mammography: Fibrocystic changes

T1-weighted sequence (precontrast) (Fig. 8.**26**)
Breast parenchyma shows hypointense signal in comparison to signal of intramammary adipose tissue. It is interspersed with varying degrees of fat tissue. Frequently seen hypointense lesions of various sizes are the representation of a cystic component.

T2-weighted sequence (Fig. 8.**27**)
Breast parenchyma with fibrocystic changes occasionally shows diffusely increased signal intensity (especially in second half of the menstrual cycle, and under hormone replacement therapy). When a cystic component is present, hyperintense lesions of various sizes may be demonstrated.

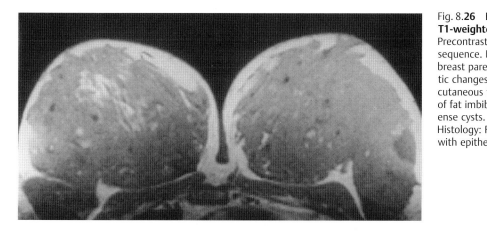

Fig. 8.**26 Fibrocystic changes in T1-weighted image.**
Precontrast T1-weighted GE sequence. Hypointense signal of breast parenchyma with fibrocystic changes in comparison to subcutaneous fat tissue. Low degree of fat imbibition. Several hypointense cysts.
Histology: Fibrocystic changes with epithelial proliferation.

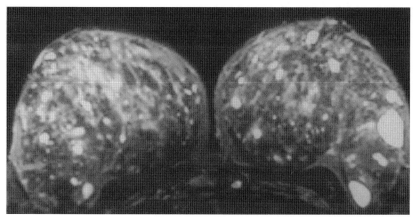

Fig. 8.**27 Fibrocystic changes in T2-weighted image.**
T2-weighted IR sequence. Hyperintense signal of breast parenchyma with fibrocystic changes. Demarcation of numerous hyperintense cysts of various sizes.
Histology: Fibrocystic changes with epithelial proliferation.

MR mammography: Fibrocystic changes

T1-weighted sequence (contrast-enhanced)

Often symmetrical distribution of areas with increased signal intensity after contrast administration (patchy, mixed patchy–diffuse, diffuse) (Figs. 8.**30**–8.**32**). Signal increases continuously within representative ROIs during the entire examination. CM uptake correlates with the degree of adenosis but not with the degree of proliferation (Figs. 8.**28** and 8.**29**). It is therefore not possible to use MR mammography to evaluate the degree of fibrocystic changes, i.e., the risk of malignant transformation (Fischer 1994; Sittek 1996). An increase of CM uptake in the first and fourth weeks of the menstrual cycle (Kuhl 1996), and under hormone replacement therapy is seen in about one-third of cases.

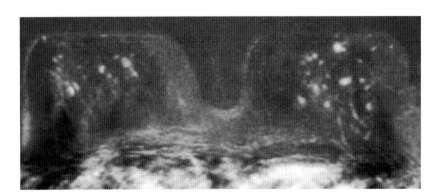

Figs. 8.**28** and 8.**29**   **Correlation between CM uptake and degree of adenosis. Comparison of images from two patients with histologically verified fibrocystic changes.**

Fig. 8.**28**   Low degree of focal adenosis showing slight, patchy contrast enhancement in MR mammography. MIP image.

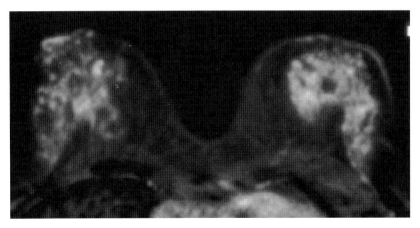

Fig. 8.**29**   Strong intramammary contrast enhancement in a patient with histologically verified, extensive areas of adenosis. MIP image.

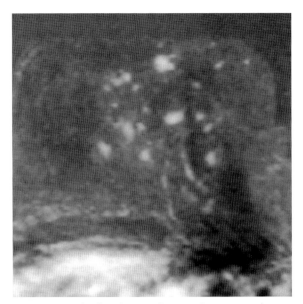

Fig. 8.**30** **Patchy distribution of areas of contrast enhancement in patient with fibrocystic changes.**
Subtraction image.

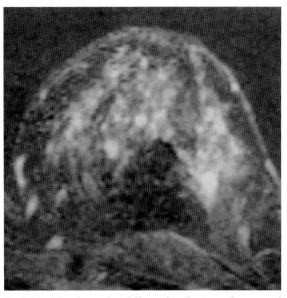

Fig. 8.**31** **Mixed patchy–diffuse distribution of areas of contrast enhancement in a patient with fibrocystic changes.**
Subtraction image.

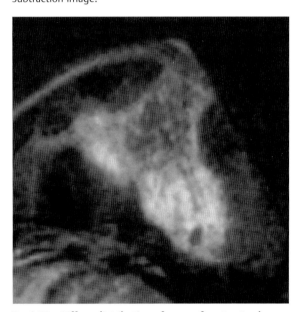

Fig. 8.**32** **Diffuse distribution of areas of contrast enhancement in a patient with fibrocystic changes.**
Subtraction image.

Adenosis

(Synonym: Adenosis mammae)

The term *adenosis* is used to describe clustered proliferations of small ductal and acinar structures in varying degrees, combined with an increase in lobular connective tissue. Adenosis of the breast is differentiated into the following types: *sclerosing adenosis* (Figs. 8.**33**, 8.**35**, and 8.**36**), *microcystic adenosis* (so-called *blunt duct adenosis*, Fig. 8.**34**), and the uncommon lesions *microglandular adenosis* and *radial scar* (synonym *radial sclerosing adenosis*, discussed separately on p. 83).

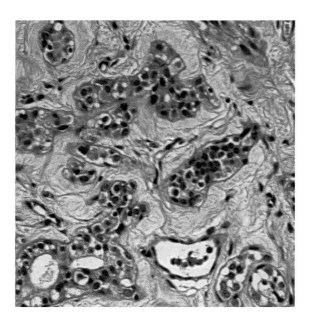

General information

Incidence:	Common benign lesion.
Age peak:	All ages.
Risk of malignant transformation:	Low (factor 2 for sclerosing adenosis).

Findings

Clinical:	Palpable mass only when area of adenosis is extensive.
Mammography:	Often presence of round, intralobular microcalcifications or milk of calcium.
Ultrasonography:	Generally no specific findings.
	Occasionally hypoechoic nodular areas within breast tissue.

Clinical significance

It is occasionally very difficult to differentiate with certainty the process creating microcalcifications.

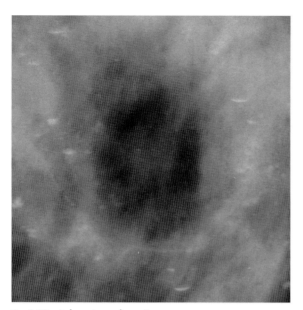

Fig. 8.**33 Sclerosing adenosis.**
Magnification mammogram shows clustered, round, and sedimented (milk of calcium) microcalcifications in a patient with histologically verified sclerosing adenosis.

 MR mammography: Adenosis

T1-weighted sequence (precontrast)
No evidence of abnormalities within the parenchyma.

T2-weighted sequence
No evidence of abnormalities within the parenchyma.

T1-weighted sequence (contrast-enhanced)
Usually strong CM uptake in focal areas of adenosis, which can show signal behavior typical for malignancy. Differentiation from carcinoma may be impossible. Occasionally branching enhancement that cannot be differentiated from an intraductal tumor. There is a correlation between fibrocystic changes with/without adenosis and the degree of CM uptake, but no corresponding correlation between contrast enhancement and the degree of epithelial proliferation (Sittek et al. 1996).

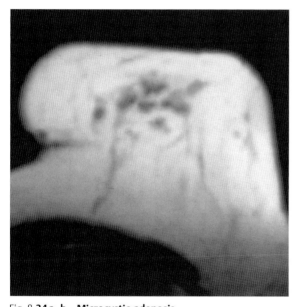 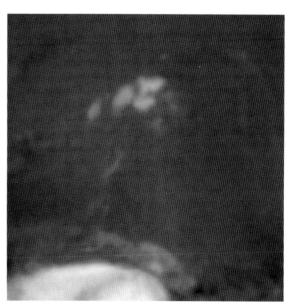

Fig. 8.**34 a, b Microcystic adenosis.**
a T1-weighted precontrast image shows normal findings with spotty distribution of parenchyma within surrounding adipose tissue.

b After contrast administration, there is evident contrast enhancement in adenotic areas (subtraction image).
Histology: Microcystic adenosis.

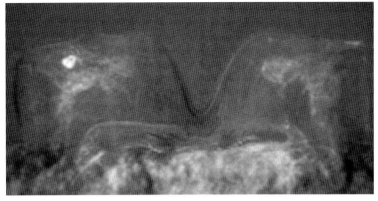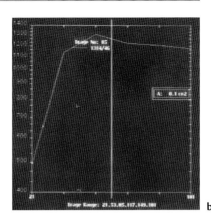

Fig. 8.35 a, b   Sclerosing adenosis.
False-positive finding in dynamic MR mammography.

a Subtraction image of both breasts demonstrates hyper-vascularized, well-circumscribed lesion in the right retro-mamillary region.

b Signal analysis shows strong initial signal increase well over 100% with postinitial plateau. Open biopsy after MR localization.

Histology: Localized area of sclerosing adenosis.

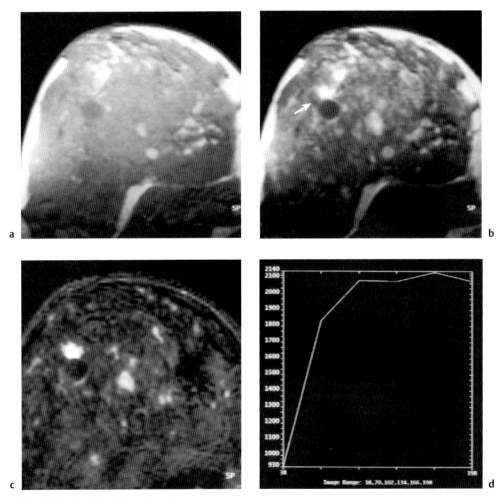

Fig. 8.36 a–d   Sclerosing adenosis.

a T1-weighted precontrast image shows few hypointense cysts.

b Patchy enhancement after contrast administration. Stellate area with CM uptake on ventral side of one cyst (arrow).

c Subtraction image depicts this lesion more clearly.

d Strong initial signal increase followed by plateau. Open biopsy after MR localization.

Histology: Focal sclerosing adenosis.

Simple Cysts

Cysts are fluid-filled round to ovoid structures that vary in size from microscopic to grossly evident as a palpable mass. Histopathology shows that the lining epithelium usually consists of two layers: an inner epithelial layer and an outer myoepithelial layer. Occasionally there may be fine intracystic septations. Cysts may occur as a singular lesion or be multiple in number and represent a typical component of fibrocystic changes (Figs. 8.**37**–8.**41**).

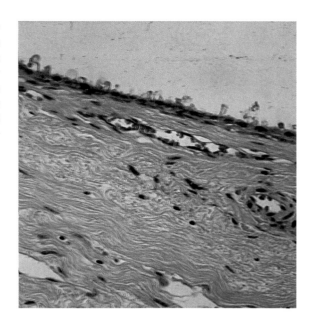

Findings

Clinical	Small cysts: usually occult
	Gross cysts: elastic, well-circumscribed and movable palpable masses, occasionally painful.
Mammography:	Small cysts: usually occult.
	Gross cysts: well-circumscribed, homogeneous round lesions. Possible halo sign.
Ultrasonography (method of choice):	Detection of small cysts from 1 mm in diameter.
	Anechoic round to ovoid lesions with smooth borders and posterior acoustic enhancement.

Clinical significance

Gross cysts can cause breast pain (mastalgia) and cn therefore be clinically relevant. In such cases, percutaneous aspiration may be performed to relieve symptoms. Small asymptomatic cysts are incidental findings.

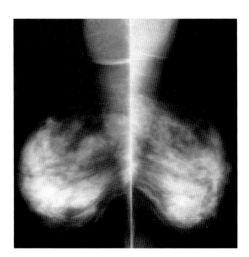

Fig. 8.**37** **Fibrocystic changes with gross cysts.**
Mammography shows multiple round densities in both breasts.

MR mammography: Simple cyst

T1-weighted sequence (precontrast)
Well-circumscribed, hypointense lesion without identifiable structure representing the cyst wall. Good demarcation of cysts located within adipose tissue. Poor demarcation of cysts located within breast parenchyma.

T2-weighted sequence
Well-circumscribed, hyperintense lesion with homogeneous internal structure. Detection possible from diameter of ~2 mm depending on matrix and FOV.

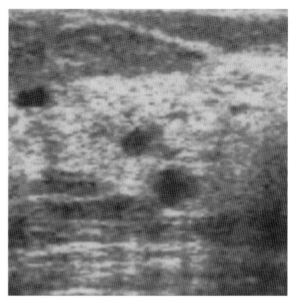

Fig. 8.**38   Fibrocystic disease.**
Ultrasonography demonstrates small cysts with posterior acoustic enhancement.

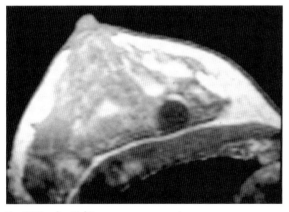

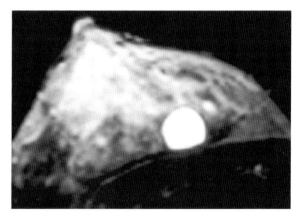

Fig. 8.**39 a, b   Solitary mammary cyst.**
a Precontrast T1-weighted GE sequence shows good demarcation of a hypointense, well-circumscribed lesion.

b In IR sequence, the well-circumscribed mammary cyst demonstrates strong hyperintense signal.

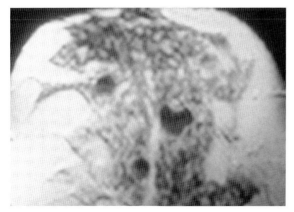

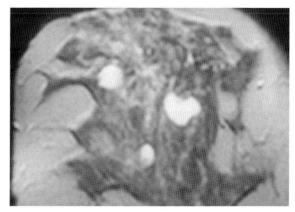

Fig. 8.**40 a, b   Multiple mammary cysts.**
a Precontrast T1-weighted GE sequence demonstrating demarcation of several hypointense lesions within parenchyma with interspersed adipose tissue.

b In the T2-weighted image, cysts show hyperintense signal.

MR mammography: Simple cyst

T1-weighted sequence (contrast-enhanced)
No significant change of existing signal intensity difference between cysts and surrounding adipose tissue after contrast administration. Improved demarcation of cystic lesions within parenchyma due to CM uptake in surrounding breast tissue. No CM uptake within simple mammary cysts.

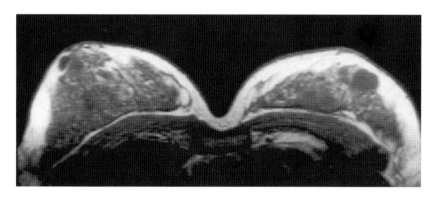

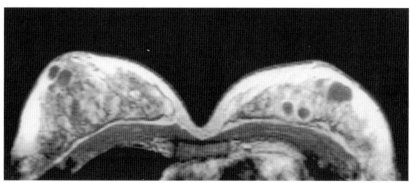

Fig. 8.**41 a, b   Mammary cysts located within breast parenchyma.**
a Precontrast T1-weighted GE sequence demonstrating the presence of a few hypointense lesions within the breast parenchyma.

b Improved demarcation of these and additional cysts after contrast administration, due to contrast enhancement of surrounding parenchyma.

Complicated Cysts

Complicated mammary cysts differ from simple mammary cysts in that inflammatory (Figs. 8.**45**, 8.**46**), hemorrhagic (Figs. 8.**43**, 8.**44**), or neoplastic (Fig. 8.**42**) changes are found within the cyst lumen or in the cyst wall.

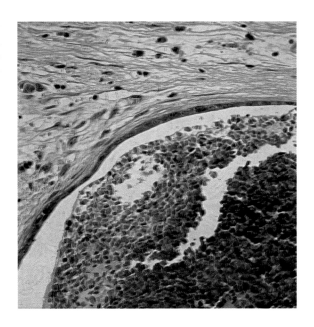

Findings

Clinical	Small cysts: usually occult.
	Gross cysts: elastic, well-circumscribed, and movable palpable masses. In rare cases differentiation from malignant tumor is dificult.
Mammography:	Findings usually as for simple cysts.
	(Partially) Ill-defined borders indicate presence of complicated cyst.
	No assessment of cyst contents is possible (exception: pneumocystogram).
Ultrasonography (method of choice):	Reliable demonstration of partial or complete wall abnormalities, atypical cyst contents, or solid intracystic tumors seen as echogenic structures.

Clinical significance

Evidence of a complicated cyst usually calls for further diagnostic evaluation by percutaneous biopsy or open biopsy.

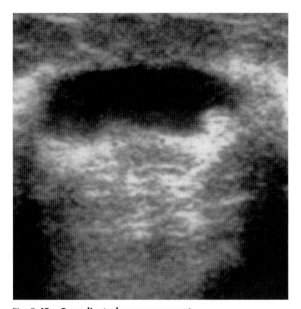

Fig. 8.42 Complicated mammary cyst.
Ultrasonography demonstrates round intraluminal lesion representing cystic carcinoma.

 MR mammography: Complicated cysts

T1-weighted sequence (precontrast)
Well-circumscribed, hypointense lesion without identifiable structure representing the cyst wall. Good demarcation of cysts located within adipose tissue. Poor demarcation between cysts and breast parenchyma. A hemorrhagic cyst (*chocolate cyst*) shows a hyperintense or isointense internal signal in comparison to the parenchymal signal, or signs of sedimentation.

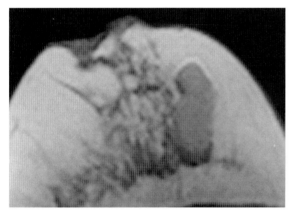

Fig. 8.43 Chocolate cyst.
Precontrast T1-weighted GE sequence shows ovoid an lesion with homogeneous hyperintense signal in comparison with breast parenchyma.

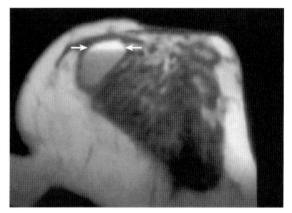

Fig. 8.44 Hemorrhagic cyst with signs of sedimentation.
Precontrast T1-weighted GE sequence shows an ovoid lesion with demonstration of blood-fluid sedimentation line (arrows). Strong hyperintense signal of sedimented blood components. In comparison with breast parenchyma, homogeneous moderately hyperintense signal of fluid. (Note: patient in prone position!)

MR mammography: Complicated cyst

T1-weighted sequence (contrast-enhanced)

Inflammation: Increased CM uptake in occasionally thickened cyst wall without enhancement of internal cyst content. When numerous cysts are present, repeat examinations often show a changing distribution of enhancing lesions.

Cave: The „ring-enhancement" seen in inflamed cysts is not a sign of malignancy. It should be assessed as a harmless side finding and therefore better termed *wall-enhancement.*

Hemorrhagic cyst: Occasional slight CM uptake in tissue surrounding cyst as a sign of reactive hyperemia.

Intracystic solid tumor: CM uptake within intracystic tumor, often showing criteria suspicious of malignancy.

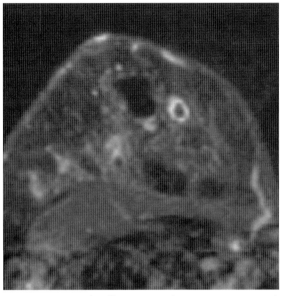

Fig. 8.**45 Cyst with inflammatory changes in patient with fibrocystic disease.**
Subtraction image with wall-enhancement of inflamed cyst and partial enhancement of another cyst wall. Several further cysts without contrast enhancement.

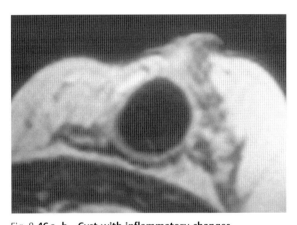 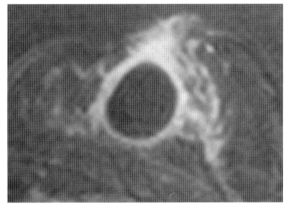

Fig. 8.**46 a, b Cyst with inflammatory changes.**
a T1-weighted GE sequence demonstrating round, retroareolar cyst with thickened cyst wall.

b Subtraction image showing strong CM uptake within thick cyst wall and portions of surrounding parenchyma.
Histology: Inflamed cyst with surrounding sclerosing adenosis.

Radial Scar

(Synonyms: sclerosing papillary proliferation, indurative mastopathy, radial sclerosing lesion)

The term *radial scar* denotes a lesion that has a stellate configuration and consists of a central, fibroelastotic (retracting) core containing glandular elements. Radiating from this core are ducts with varying degrees of epithelial hyperplasia and papillomatosis (Figs. 8.**47**–8.**50**). Sclerosing adenosis and apocrine metaplasia are frequently found in close proximity.

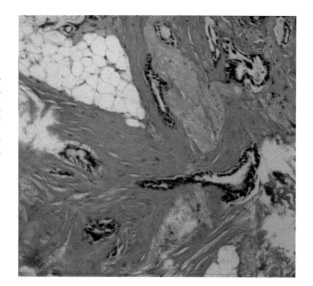

General information

Incidence:	Rare (no proven data).
Age peak:	All ages.
Risk of malignant transformation:	Transitional states to tubular breast cancer have been described. Studies verify its significance as a precancerosis.

Findings

Clinical:	Usually no palpable mass in correlation. Usually an incidental finding on mammography or in excised breast tissue. Multiple occurrence has been described.
Mammography:	Soft-tissue density with scirrhous configuration. Typically <1 cm in diameter (>1 cm: „complex sclerosing lesions").
Ultrasonography:	Occasionally hypoechoic stellate lesion.

Clinical significance

It is usually not possible to differentiate radial scars from scirrhous carcinomas. Local excision is the treatment of choice.

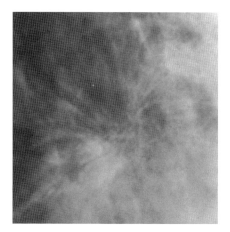

Fig. 8.**47   Radial scar.**
Spot compression mammography shows typical stellate structure with central retraction.

MR mammography: Radial scar

T1-weighted sequence (precontrast)
Stellate lesion with signal intensity equivalent to that of parenchyma. When located within parenchyma it is therefore difficult or impossible to identify. Good detectability within adipose tissue.

T2-weighted sequence
No characteristic finding.

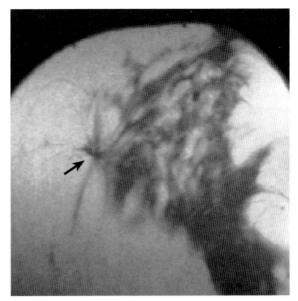

Fig. 8.**48   Radial scar.**
T1-weighted precontrast image with demonstration of stellate, hypointense lesion within adipose tissue (arrow).
Histology: Radial scar.

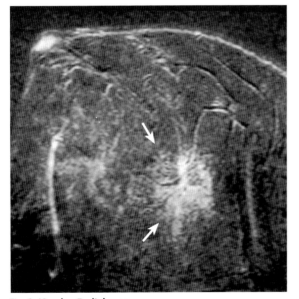

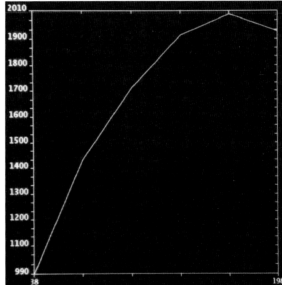

Fig. 8.**49 a, b   Radial scar.**
a Subtraction image demonstrating hypervascularized area with partially stellate borders in the central region of the right breast.

b Moderate initial contrast enhancement with continuous post-initial increase in the signal intensity curve.
Histology: Radial scar.

MR mammography: Radial scar

T1-weighted sequence (contrast-enhanced)
Slight to moderate CM uptake within the stellate lesion. Generally unspecific signal intensity curve. Taking all diagnostic criteria into consideration, the constellation of findings is often suspicious for malignancy.

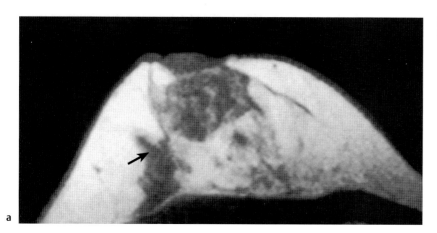

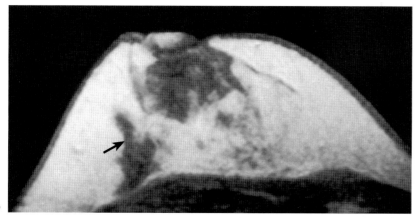

Fig. 8.50 a–d   Radial scar.
a The precontrast image shows a very discrete stellate structure (arrow).

b Strong enhancement after contrast administration.
c Better detectability in subtraction image.
d Moderate initial contrast enhancement with postinitial plateau in the signal intensity curve.
Histology (after preoperative stereotactic localization): Radial scar.

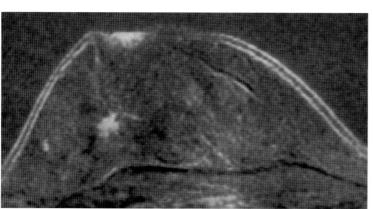

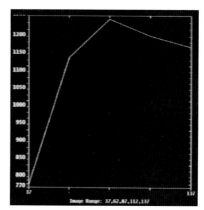

Hamartoma

(Figuratively: „Breast within the breast"; Kronsbein and Bässler 1982)

Hamartomas of the breast are well-defined lesions with organoid structure and fissurelike or pseudocapsular borders. They are composed of adipose tissue, fibrous stroma, and parenchyma (with or without cystic inclusions) in varying proportions (Figs. 8.**51**–8.**53**).

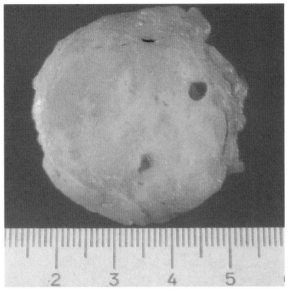

(Courtesy of Prof. Dr. R. Bässler, Fulda)

General information

Incidence:	Rare (1:1000).
Age peak:	40–60 years.
Risk of malignant transformation:	No increased risk.

Findings

Clinical:	Occult (if high lipomatous component).
	Palpable mass (if high fibrotic component).
Mammography (method of choice):	Well-circumscribed lesion with lipomatous inclusions.
	Halo sign due to compression of surrounding tissue.
Ultrasonography:	Well-circumscribed lesion with hypoechoic inclusions.

Clinical significance

Incidental finding without therapeutic consequences if no signs of malignancy are present.

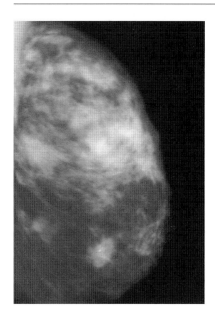

 MR mammography: Hamartoma

T1-weighted sequence (precontrast)
Well-circumscribed round, oval or lobulated lesion. Pseudocapsular demarcation and organoid internal structures (parenchymal components with intermediary signal intensity, lipomatous components with hyperintense signal, and cystic components with hypointense signal).

T2-weighted sequence
Well-circumscribed round, oval, or lobulated lesion. Pseudocapsular demarcation and organoid internal structures (parenchymal and lipomatous components with intermediary signal intensity, cystic components with hyperintense signal).

◁ Fig. 8.**51 Hamartoma.**
Conventional mammography shows a well-circumscribed lesion with both lipomatous and parenchymatous components in axillary tail of breast.

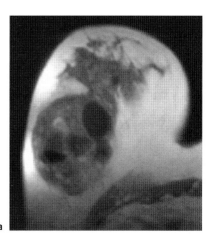

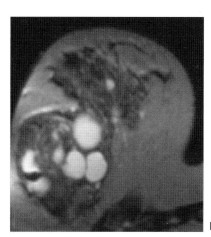

Fig. 8.**52 a, b Hamartoma.**
a T1-weighted sequence shows a well-circumscribed lesion with inhomogeneous internal structure (parenchyma, fat, cysts).
b T2-weighted sequence demonstrates strong signal intensity of cystic internal structures. Histology: Hamartoma.

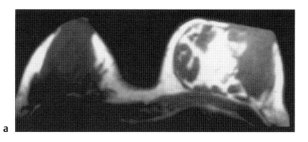

 MR mammography: Hamartoma

T1-weighted sequence (contrast-enhanced)
No CM uptake in lipomatous and cystic portions of hamartoma. Dependent upon vascularization, no to strong contrast enhancement in parenchymatous portions of hamartoma, usually with continuous postinitial signal increase.

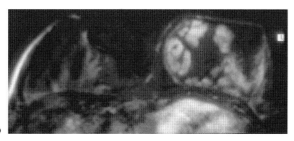

Fig. 8.**53 a, b Hamartoma.**
a T1-weighted sequence shows a hamartoma with both parenchymatous and lipomatous components occupying the entire left breast.
b Subtraction image demonstrates strong enhancement in nonlipomatous hamartoma components.
Histology: Hamartoma.

Acute Mastitis

The term *acute mastitis* is used to describe an infection of the breast with primary canalicular ascending and secondary interstitial spread. Mastitis occurring during the lactational period is designated **puerperal mastitis**. If it occurs outside this period, it is called **nonpuerperal mastitis** (Figs. 8.**54**–8.**56**). Conditions that predispose to nonpuerperal mastitis are immunosuppressive therapy and diabetes.

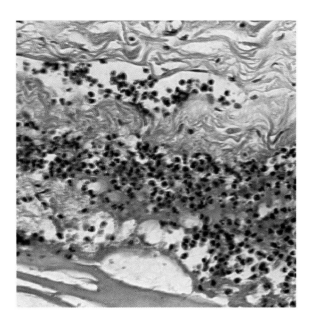

General information

Incidence:	Very rare.
Age peak:	All ages.
Complications:	Abscess or fistula formation.

Findings

Clinical ethod of choice):	Hyperthermia, erythema, pain (classical triad indicating inflammation), and swelling of breast. Lymphadenitis, abscess formation, skin thickening. Fever and elevated laboratory parameters indicating inflammation.
Exfoliative cytology and/ or percutaneous biopsy (method of choice):	Isolation of cultured organisms.
Mammography:	Diffuse reduction of transparency (indistinct structures) in comparison to contralateral breast; skin thickening.
Ultrasonography:	Increased echogeneity of subcutaneous structures, skin thickening.

Clinical significance

Clinical examination and breast imaging techniques do not allow a reliable differentiation between nonpuerperal mastitis and inflammatory breast cancer. Failure to respond to antibiotic therapy therefore makes it necessary to perform a biopsy to rule out malignancy.

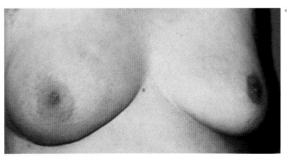

◁ Fig. 8.**54**   **Mastitis.**
Clinical presentation of nonpuerperal mastitis with erythema and swelling of the right breast.

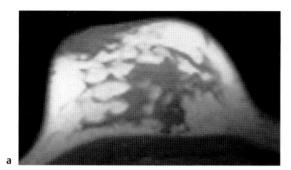

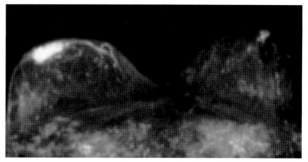

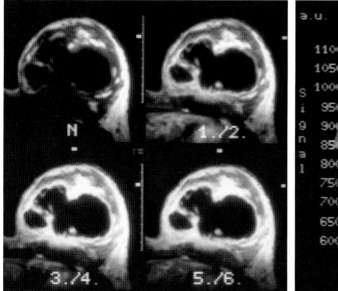

Fig. 8.55 a–c   Acute nonpuerperal mastitis.

a T1-weighted precontrast image shows a circumscribed area of low signal intensity in the right retroareolar and periareolar region.

b The MIP technique documents an area of hypervascularization in this area (right breast). Physiological enhancement of the nipple on the left.

c Signal analysis shows strong initial contrast enhancement with postinitial plateau.
Histology: Acute mastitis.

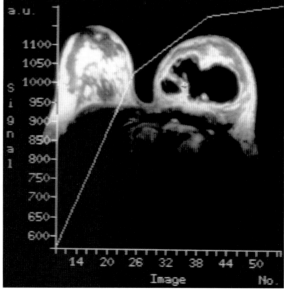

Fig. 8.56 a, b   Puerperal mastitis with breast abscess formation.

a T1-weighted precontrast image (N) shows extensive fluid accumulation within the entire left breast in patient with intramammary abscesses. After contrast administration, increasing enhancement in the abscess wall and surrounding parenchyma (1–6 minutes).

b Signal intensity curve shows moderate initial contrast enhancement with continuous postinitial increase.
Histology: Mastitis with abscess formation.

Chronic Nonpuerperal Mastitis

Chronic nonpuerperal mastitis is an aseptic inflammatory process in and around the terminal ducts and lobuli of the breast (Figs. 8.**57**–8.**59**). Three forms of mastitis are classified according to their histology and pathogenesis: **galactophoritic**, **granulomatous**, and **lobular**. The galactophoritic and granulomatous (obliterative) forms of mastitis are characterized by retention of secretions, duct ectasia, and periductal mastitis. Lobular mastitis is also destructive and granulomatous. In the final stage of periductal mastitis, one typically finds hyaline changes of the ducts with calcification.

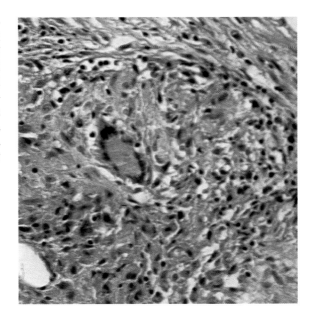

General information	
Incidence:	5–25% of all women (depending on definition). In daily praxis more likely <5%.
Distribution:	Often bilateral.
Age peak:	30–90 years (maximum 40–49 years).
Complications:	Fistula formation, abscess formation (very rare).

Findings	
Clinical:	Painful symptoms are rare. Nipple discharge (rarely sanguineous); less common are nipple retraction or periareolar fistulas.
Mammography:	Dilated retromamillary ducts. Microcalcifications rare in early stages. In later stages, typical spherical and tubular calcifications with lucent centers, and linear microcalcifications with orientation toward the nipple.
Galactography:	Subareolar ductal ectasia; CM depicts cystic dilatation of ductal structures.
Ultrasonography:	Hypoechoic tubular structures in retromamillary region (ductal ectasia). Occasionally hypoechoic (granulomas) or anechoic (cystic) areas.

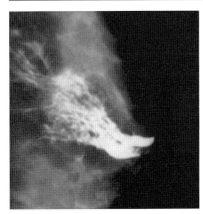

Fig. 8.**57**   **Duct ectasia.**
Galactography demonstrates dilated ducts.

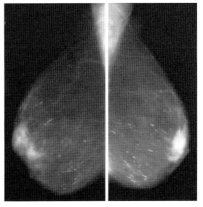

Fig. 8.**58**   **Plasma cell mastitis.**
Mammography demonstrates typical linear calcifications.

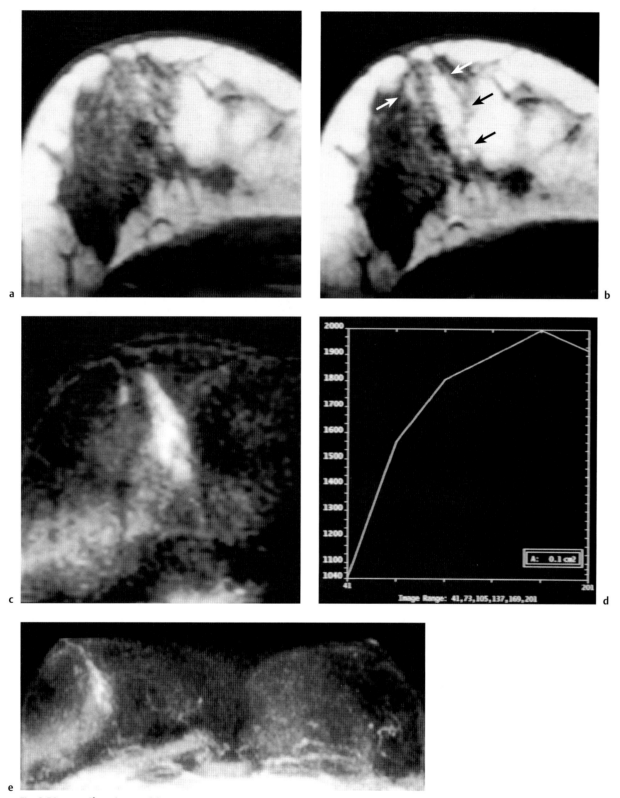

Fig. 8.**59 a–e   Chronic mastitis.**
a Normal depiction of right breast in T1-weighted precontrast image.
b Subareolar segmental enhancement after contrast administration (arrows).
c Documentation in subtraction image.

d Documentation in MIP technique.
e Moderate initial contrast enhancement. Signal maximum in fourth measurement after contrast administration.

Histology: Chronic mastitis along major mammary ducts.

Intramammary Lymph Nodes

Intramammary lymph nodes are those found within the breast parenchyma. They do not differ histologically from lymph nodes found in other locations (Figs. 8.**60**– 8.**62**).

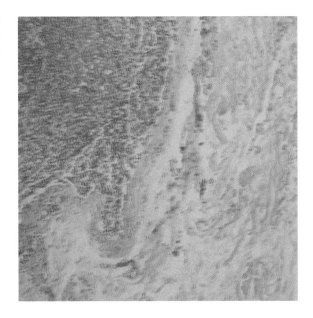

General information

Incidence:	Common physiological finding.
Age peak:	All ages.

Findings

Clinical:	Generally occult.
Mammography:	Oval, occasionally round, well-circumscribed lesion.
	Characteristic radiolucent (fat) area in center or periphery.
Ultrasonography:	Hyperechoic center and hypoechoic peripheral structure (identical to axillary lymph nodes).

Clinical significance

Intramammary lymph nodes are usually a harmless incidental finding. Intramammary lymph node metastases are rare. According to the TNM classification, they are classed as axillary lymph nodes.

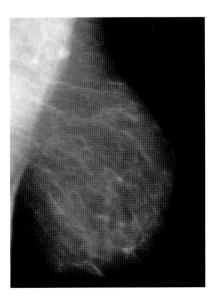

Fig. 8.**60**   **Intramammary lymph node.**
Mammography shows an oval, well-circumscribed mass in typical localization ventral to the pectoral muscle.

MR mammography: Lymph nodes

T1-weighted sequence (precontrast)
No demarcation when located within parenchyma. Lymph nodes in more common extraparenchymal localization within adipose tissue are seen as oval, well-circumscribed, hypointense lesion. Central hyperintense areas are characteristic.

T2-weighted sequence
No characteristic findings.

T1-weighted sequence (contrast-enhanced)
Normally no or only slight contrast enhancement within bland lymph nodes. Lymph nodes showing reactive inflammatory changes (especially several weeks to months after a surgical procedure) can, however, sometimes demonstrate an extremely strong contrast enhancement displaying signs of malignancy (e.g., wash-out phenomenon).

Cave: A lymph node with a central fat inclusion and inflammatory changes can produce an image simulating ring-enhancement.

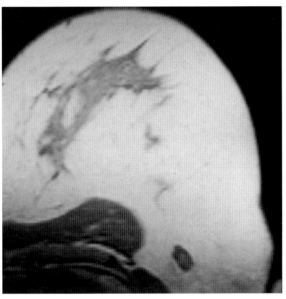

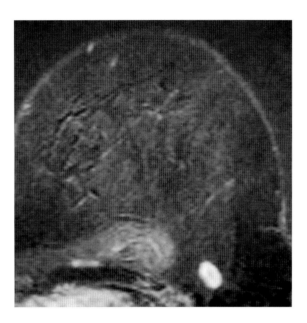

Fig. 8.**61 a, b   Lymph node in typical location.**
a T1-weighted precontrast image showing a well-circumscribed lesion ventral to the pectoral muscle. Central fat inclusion.

b Ringlike enhancement after contrast administration results from central fat without CM uptake and nonspecific inflammation of lymphatic tissue.

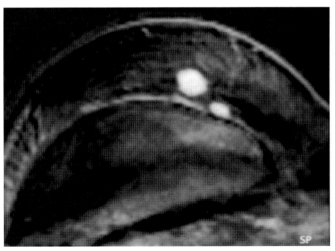

Fig. 8.**62 a, b   Intramammary lymph node.**
a Strong contrast enhancement in two intramammary lymph nodes with inflammatory changes after mastectomy and reconstructive surgery one year earlier.

b Strong initial contrast enhancement with postinitial plateau. Histology: Lymphadenitis. No malignancy.

Fat necrosis

(Synonym: liponecrosis microcystica calcificata)

Fat necrosis is a localized area of dead adipose tissue characterized by morphological changes resulting from progressive enzymatic degradation. Leukocytic and histiocytic infiltrates are encountered in new areas of fat necrosis. Gradually, well-vascularized granulation tissue then develops. The transformation into scar tissue is usually complete within a matter of weeks. The coalescence of liquefied adipose tissue can lead to formation of so-called *oil cysts* (Figs. 8.**63**–8.**66**).

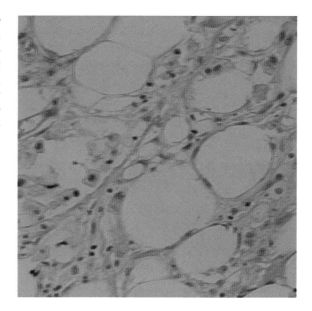

General information

Etiology:	Posttraumatic (injury, surgery, needle biopsy), inflammation, foreign body reaction (silicone, paraffin).
Risk of malignant transformation:	No increased risk.

Findings

Clinical:	Usually occult. Occasionally presence of painless mass or skin thickening. Personal history: biopsy? surgery? Inspection: visible scars?
Mammography:	Fresh: ill-defined area of increased density. Later: improving demarcation of density. *Oil cysts*: rounded, centrally radiolucent lesions possibly containing bizarre or rim calcifications.
Ultrasonography:	Great variations: from round, well-circumscribed lesions to lesions showing characteristics of malignancy.

Clinical significance

Occasionally, fat necrosis can be very difficult to differentiate from breast cancer, i.e., cancer relapse, using breast imaging techniques.

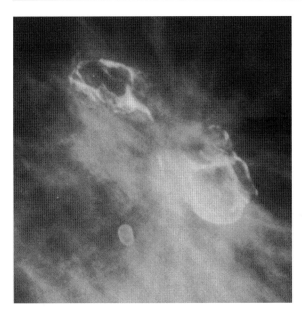

Fig. 8.**63 Fat necrosis.**
Mammography shows bizarre macrocalcifications in postoperative fat necrosis.

 MR mammography: Fat necrosis

T1-weighted sequence (precontrast)
Signal intensity equivalent to that of parenchyma. Possible postoperative susceptibility artifacts due to electrocauterization. When oil cysts are present, rounded lesions with hyperintense (fat-equivalent) signal. Possible signal loss due to macrocalcifications.

T2-weighted sequence
Fresh fat necrosis results in ill-defined, hyperintense areas due to reactive edema. Later, when oil cysts are present, depiction of rounded lesions with central, fat-equivalent signal intensity. Otherwise no characteristic changes after six months.

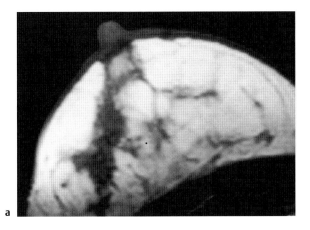

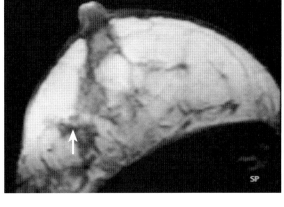

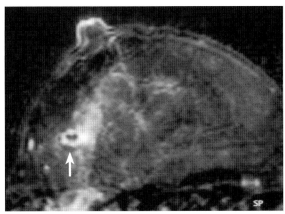

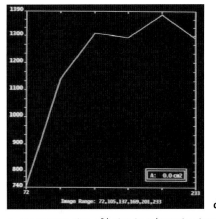

Fig. 8. **64 a–d Fresh fat necrosis.**
Postlumpectomy patient.
a Normal T1-weighted precontrast examination.
b Regional enhancement in parenchyma after contrast administration. Hypervascularized area with ringlike enhancement in lateral portion of breast (arrow).

c Documentation of lesion in subtraction image (arrow).
d Signal curve analysis shows moderate initial signal enhancement with postinitial plateau. This lesion was excised simultaneously with tumor recurrence at another location (not shown).
Histology: Fat necrosis.

MR mammography: Fat necrosis

T1-weighted sequence (contrast-enhanced)
In the early phase, when capillary sprouting takes place (first six months after trauma/surgery), fat necrosis presents as a localized but not sharply defined area with increased CM uptake. The initial signal enhancement is usually moderate, the post-initial signal increase is typically continuous, more rarely a plateau. In the late phase (more than six months), normally no areas with increased enhancement are present unless there is an additional inflammatory component.

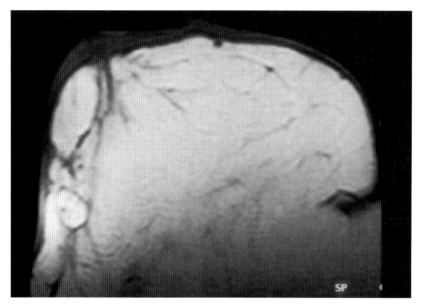

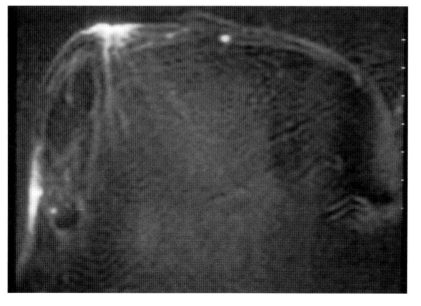

Fig. 8.65 a, b   Fat necrosis with oil cyst.

a T1-weighted precontrast image shows a signal-intense lesion corresponding to a known oil cyst. The lower peripheral signal is due to rim calcifications. Additional aspect: Skin thickening due to radiotherapy after lumpectomy 14 months earlier.

b No relevant enhancement after contrast administration in oil cyst location. Localized enhancement in the vein lateral to the oil cyst, in the right mammillary region, and in the vessel cross section medial to the nipple.

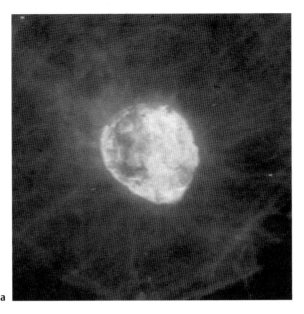

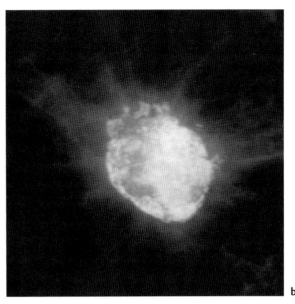

a

b

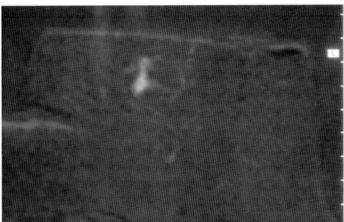

d

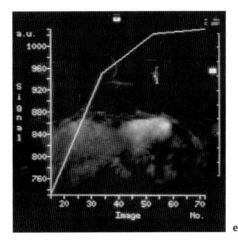

e

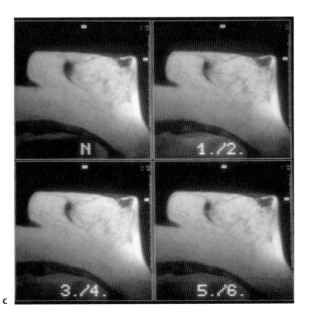

c

Fig. 8.66 a–e   Fat necrosis with additional focal mastitis.
a Bizarre macrocalcification in fat necrosis two years after lumpectomy and radiotherapy (selective magnification of mammographic image).
b Destruction of upper pole of macrocalcification and increasing development of spiculated, adjoining density in mammography one year later.
c Dynamic MR mammography demonstrates signal-free lesion corresponding to macrocalcification. Discretely increased peripheral enhancement.
d Documentation of peripheral CM uptake in subtraction image.
e The signal intensity curve shows slight initial contrast enhancement with postinitial signal increase.
Histology: Fat necrosis with peripheral focal inflammatory component.

Postoperative Changes

Seroma

A seroma is a localized collection of wound serum in the tissues, for example, after surgery (Figs. 8.**67** and 8.**68**). The diagnostic method of choice is ultrasonography.

 MR mammography: Seroma

T1-weighted sequence (precontrast)
More or less circumscribed area usually demonstrating a slightly hypointense signal in comparison to surrounding parenchyma.

T2-weighted sequence
Hyperintense areas of fluid retention within parenchyma.

T1-weighted sequence (contrast-enhanced)
Immediately after surgery usually slight, after several days stronger CM uptake in immediately surrounding areas of seroma.

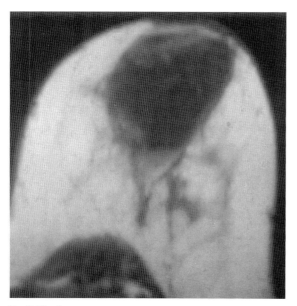

Fig. 8.**67** **Seroma.**
T1-weighted precontrast examination shows an oval lesion of low signal intensity in retromamillary region after surgery. Few intraluminal parenchymal areas. No signal enhancement after contrast administration (not shown).

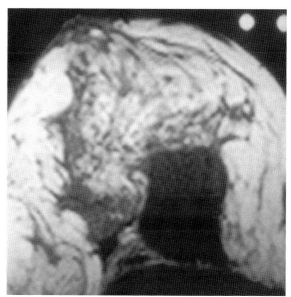

Fig. 8.**68** **Seroma.**
T1-weighted precontrast examination shows a spindle-shaped lesion of low signal intensity close to the chest wall after surgery. No signal enhancement after contrast administration (not shown).

Hematoma

A breast hematoma is an intramammary hemorrhage, for example, postoperatively (Fig. 8.**69**). The diagnostic method of choice is ultrasonography.

 MR mammography: Hematoma

T1-weighted sequence (precontrast)
A hematoma shows a typical signal intensity, as in other regions of the body, depending on the time elapsed since its development. A fresh hemorrhage demonstrates a homogeneous high signal intensity, possibly with signs of sedimentation. A subacute hemorrhage shows a low internal signal with a peripheral ring of high signal intensity.

T2-weighted sequence
A hematoma shows a typical signal intensity, as in other regions of the body, depending on the time elapsed since its development. A fresh hemorrhage demonstrates a homogeneous low signal intensity, a subacute hemorrhage low signal intensity with a peripheral ring of low signal intensity.

T1-weighted sequence (contrast-enhanced)
Diffuse reactive CM uptake in parenchyma surrounding hematoma. Initial contrast enhancement in this area is slight to moderate, usually showing a continuous postinitial signal increase. No CM uptake within hematoma.

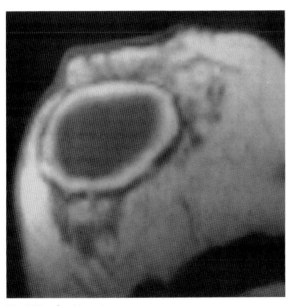
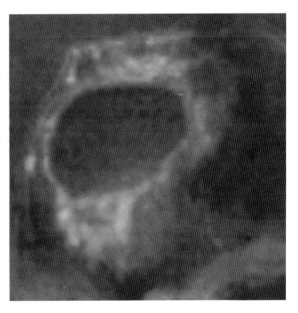

Fig. 8.**69 a, b** **Hematoma.**

a T1-weighted precontrast image shows subacute intramammary hematoma. Peripheral hyperintense ring due to conversion of methemoglobin to deoxyhemoglobin.

b Subtraction image shows reactive contrast enhancement in areas immediately surrounding hematoma. No enhancement within hematoma itself.

Abscess

A breast abscess is a localized intramammary collection of pus in a cavity formed by an inflammatory disintegration of tissue, for example, postoperatively (Fig. 8.**70**). The diagnostic method of choice is ultrasonography.

 MR mammography: Abscess

T1-weighted sequence (precontrast)

Round or ovoid, less commonly polygonal, lesion with hyperintense signal due to high protein content (in comparison to parenchymal signal intensity).

T2-weighted sequence

Circumscribed round or ovoid, less commonly polygonal, lesion with high signal intensity. Occasionally increased perifocal signal intensity as an indication of reactive hyperemia. Otherwise usually no existing criteria to differentiate abscess from seroma.

T1-weighted sequence (contrast-enhanced)

No CM uptake within fluid contents. Strong contrast enhancement in abscess wall, seen as wall-enhancement (differential diagnosis: carcinoma).

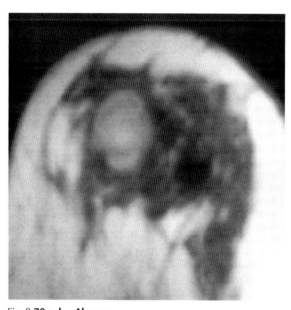 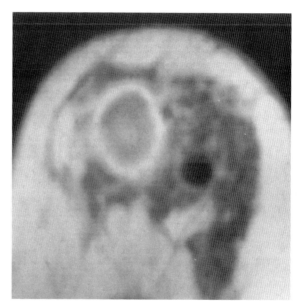

Fig. 8.**70 a, b   Abscess.**

a T1-weighted precontrast image shows an oval, hyperintense lesion within parenchyma. Hypointense cysts are incidental findings.

b T1-weighted image three minutes after contrast administration shows unchanged signal intensity in abscess fluid. Prominent ringlike enhancement as a result of CM uptake in abscess wall. Demarcation of cysts due to physiological contrast enhancement within parenchyma.

Scar tissue

Scar tissue is mostly composed of collagen fibers with a few fibrocytes and some blood vessels. In the course of the wound healing, scar tissue develops from granulation tissue ca. 3–6 months after tissue injury (e.g., surgery, trauma) (Fig. 8.**71**).

 MR mammography: Scar tissue

T1-weighted sequence (precontrast)
Usually an ill-defined or stellate structure with low signal intensity. Difficult to detect when located within parenchyma. If located within adipose tissue, can be identified as high-contrast figure.

T2-weighted sequence
Usually an ill-defined or stellate structure with low signal intensity.

T1-weighted sequence (contrast-enhanced)
No CM uptake. Only if focal inflammation is present can smaller hypervascularized areas that overlap the scar tissue be demonstrated. These show a moderate initial contrast enhancement and continuous postinitial signal increase, rarely a postinitial plateau.

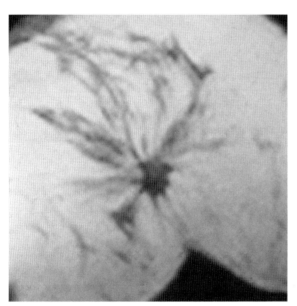 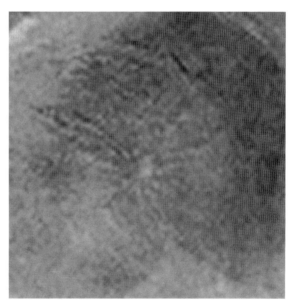

Fig. 8.**71 a, b Scar tissue.**
a T1-weighted precontrast image shows a stellate, hypointense lesion within surrounding adipose tissue. Note long radial spiculations.

b Subtraction image shows no enhancement within scar tissue.

Changes Following Radiotherapy

Radiation therapy after breast-conserving surgery for breast cancer usually requires the administration of a total dose in the range of 60 Gy, applied in fractions of 2–2.5 Gy. In addition, a boost of 10 Gy is applied to the tumor site. The acute reaction in the breast to radiotherapy is usually hyperthermia, edema, and a feeling of increased pressure. Although this phase usually lasts only several weeks, it can occasionally take months for symptoms to decrease. This recovery interval is very variable. Possible late changes include hyperpigmentation of the skin, increased breast firmness, and breast deformation (Figs. 8.**72** and 8.**73**).

 MR mammography: The irradiated breast

T1-weighted sequence (precontrast)
Skin thickening (asymmetry!), occasionally lasting several years.

T2-weighted sequence
Asymmetry with pronounced increase of signal intensity in the parenchyma of the irradiated breast, usually lasting several years.

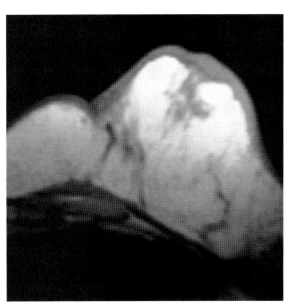
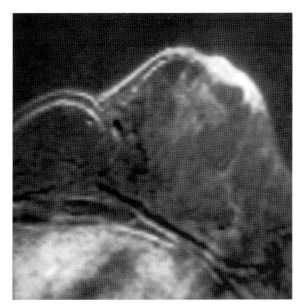

Fig. 8.**72 a, b   Irradiated breast.**
a T1-weighted precontrast examination six months after the end of radiotherapy following breast-conserving surgery. Note prominent skin thickening.

b Subtraction image after contrast administration shows prominent enhancement in skin; lesser enhancement is also seen in parenchyma.

MR mammography: The irradiated breast

T1-weighted sequence (contrast-enhanced)
Regional or diffuse enhancement of irradiated parenchyma and skin thickening. Great interindividual variability with changes lasting from three months to two years after radiotherapy. Sig-nal intensity curve in areas of increased CM up-take demonstrates moderate initial signal en-hancement (<100%), and continuous postinitial signal increase or plateau. No wash-out. Enhance-ment within the skin often seen as double line structure (railroad track).

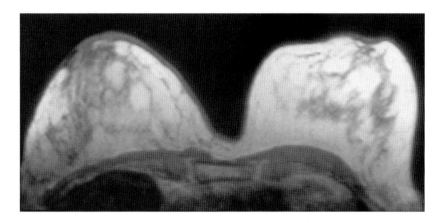

Fig. 8.73 a–c Irradiated breast.
MR mammography 18 months after lumpectomy for breast cancer in the right breast and sub-sequent radiotherapy.
a T1-weighted precontrast image showing skin thickening.

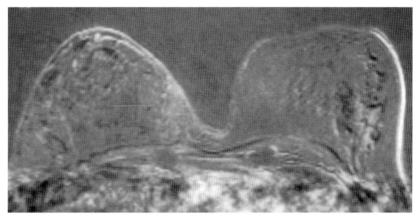

b No significant enhancement in parenchyma after contrast ad-ministration. Persistence of double line enhancement in the periareolar region of skin thickening in the right breast. Motion artifacts in the lateral portion of the left breast.

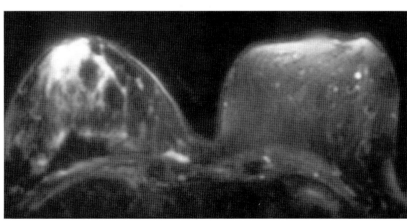

c T2-weighted image shows pro-nounced signal increase in parenchyma of the right breast.

9 Malignant Changes

Intraductal Tumor Forms

Ductal Carcinoma In Situ (DCIS)

Ductal carcinoma in situ is characterized by a proliferation of tumor cells confined to the ductal units of the breast without light-microscopic evidence of invasion through the basement membrane into the surrounding stroma.

The term ductal carcinoma in situ encompasses a pathologically heterogeneous group of lesions. The **comedo type** of DCIS is characterized by prominent necrosis in the center of the involved ducts. The **noncomedo type** of DCIS is further differentiated into *solid*, *cribriform*, *micropapillary*, *papillary*, and *clinging* types with different histological patterns (Figs. 9.**1**–9.**5**). Coexistence of several patterns in any one case is common.

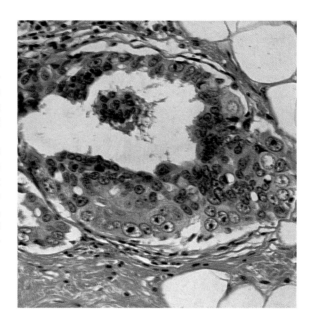

General information

Incidence:	In screening 20%. Most commonly comedo type-50% of all DCIS.
Age peak:	40-60 years
Multifocality:	Approximately 30%.
Bilaterality:	Not significantly increased.
Risk of malignant transformation:	Up to 50% for comedo type DCIS; lower for noncomedo types.

Findings

Clinical:	Often occult. Palpable mass in ~10% of cases. Occasionally pathological nipple discharge or visible changes.
Mammography (method of choice):	Suspicious microcalcifications in ~70% of cases (more common in comedo than in noncomedo type DCIS). Magnification mammography occasionally helpful. Rare appearance as spiculated mass (~20%).
Ultrasonography:	Usually no characteristic findings.

Clinical significance

The heterogeneous group of DCIS lesions are considered to be precancerous lesions, yet not all patients with DCIS will develop an invasive cancer in the ipsilateral breast. The full extent of DCIS lesions is often difficult to estimate with imaging techniques. The recommended treatment is still a matter of controversy.

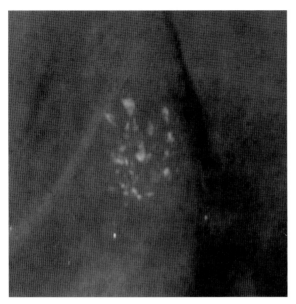

Fig. 9.**1 Mammography depicting DCIS.**
Clustered, pleomorphic microcalcifications.
Histology: Comedo type of ductal carcinoma in situ.

 MR mammography: DCIS

T1-weighted sequence (precontrast)
Isointense signal behavior in comparison to surrounding breast parenchyma. No specific changes
indicating the presence of a DCIS lesion. The spatial resolution of MR mammography does not
allow the depiction of microcalcifications.

T2-weighted sequence
No specific changes.

T1-weighted sequence (contrast-enhanced)
Branching, less commonly spiculated or round,
hypervascularized lesion with ill-defined margins. No ring-enhancement. Analysis of the signal
intensity curve shows characteristics typical of
malignancy in 50% of cases. In 40% the signal
analysis is unspecific. In 10% there is no CM uptake. The sensitivity of MR mammography is
slightly higher for comedo-type DCIS than for
noncomedo types.

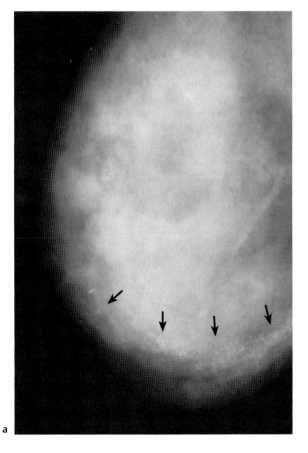

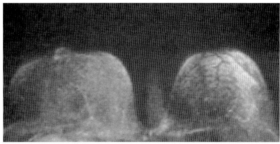

Fig. 9.**2 a, b Extensive DCIS.**
False-negative finding in MR mammography.
a Mammography shows segmental distribution of microcalcifications in the caudal portion of the right breast (arrows).
b No findings in corresponding MR mammography after contrast administration (MIP image).
Histology: Comedo-type DCIS extending over an area of ~4 ×
6 cm.

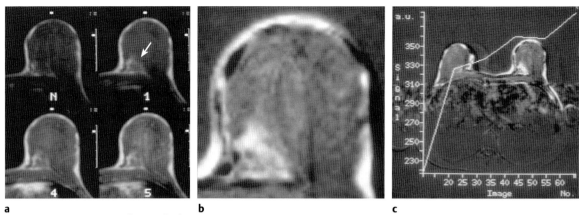

a   b   c

Fig. 9.3 a–c   DCIS; unspecific MRI findings.

Corresponding mammogram shows clustered, pleomorphic microcalcifications in upper inner quadrant of left breast (see Fig. 9.**1**).

a MR mammography shows branching area of contrast enhancement (arrow).

b Documentation of findings in subtraction image despite motion artifacts.

c Signal analysis shows no characteristics of malignancy.

Histology: Noncomedo type of DCIS.

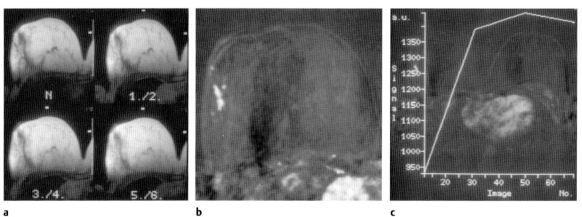

a   b   c

Fig. 9.4 a–c   DCIS; suspicious MRI findings.

Corresponding mammogram shows microcalcifications with segmental distribution (no image).

a Dynamic MR mammography shows linear contrast enhancement.

b Documentation of findings in subtraction image.

c Signal analysis shows moderate initial contrast enhancement with postinitial plateau.

Histology: Noncomedo type of DCIS.

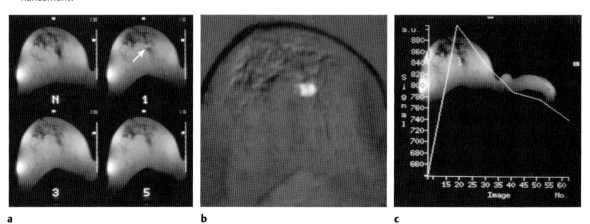

a   b   c

Fig. 9.5 a–c   DCIS; MRI findings suspicious of malignancy.

Corresponding mammogram shows microcalcifications with clustered distribution (no image).

a Dynamic MR mammography shows two adjacent, partially ill-defined hypervascularized lesions (arrow).

b Subtraction image.

c Signal analysis shows slight initial contrast enhancement with postinitial "wash-out".

Histology: Comedo type of DCIS.

Results of Literature Survey

It can be assumed that the sensitivity of dynamic MR mammography for the detection of DCIS is of the order of 50–60%. In a number of patients with in situ cancer, no contrast enhancement can be detected. In other patients one finds hypervascularized areas with unspecific signal intensity curves that do not allow the diagnosis of cancer to be made prospectively. That ductal carcinoma in situ cannot be reliably detected in MR mammography is not due to the limited spatial resolution but more to the fact that these tumors do not demonstrate a high level of neoangiogenesis. At least a proportion of DCIS lesions are apparently supplied with their growth requirements by diffusion over a long period before pathological tumor vessels develop and visualization in MR mammography becomes possible.

Published data on the sensitivity of MR mammography in detecting DCIS vary greatly depending upon the selection criteria and evaluation modalities (Table 9.1).

On the other hand, there are reports of DCIS lesions that have been detected solely in MR mammography.

These are apparently lesions that have formed pathological tumor vessels at an early stage in their development, or DCIS lesions with incipient invasion, i.e. a microinvasive component, resulting in a detectable contrast enhancement. In our experience, the proportion of DCIS lesions seen only in MR mammography is ~5% of all additionally detected carcinomas.

The detection of an intraductal tumor component is of great importance in the preoperative staging before breast conserving therapy (see Chapter 11). In one of our own studies, intraductal tumor spreading out from the primary tumor, i.e., an extensive intraductal component (EIC), was detected in 8% of preoperatively performed MR mammography examinations. In these cases the previously performed x-ray mammography and ultrasonography examinations had not indicated the presence of an EIC (Fischer et al. 1999). Other authors have reported a sensitivity of MR mammography for the detection of EIC of the order of 80–90% (Mumtaz et al. 1997; Soderstrom et al. 1996).

Table 9.**1**   DCIS: Sensitivity in MR Mammography

Author (year)	DCIS (C/NC)	False Findings in MRI
Boné et al. (1996)	17 (n.s.)	18% false-negative
Fischer et al. (1996)	35 (21/14)	29% without CE
		29% unspecific CE
Gilles et al. (1995)	36 (24/12)[1]	6% without early enhancement
Orel et al. (1997)	13 (6/7)	23% false-negative
Rieber et al. (1997)	7 (n.s.)[2]	100% false-negative
Soderstrom et al. (1997)	11 (n.s.)[3]	0% false-negative
Tesoro-Tess et al. (1995)	6 (3/3)	50% false-negative
Viehweg et al. (1999)	37 (n.s.)[1]	50% atypical findings

C, comedo type; NC, noncomedo type; n.s., not stated.
[1] 1/3 of these with microinvasive component.
[2] Strong selection of patient population.
[3] Six of these with microinvasive component.

Lobular Carcinoma In Situ (LCIS)

Lobular carcinoma in situ is characterized by a proliferation of tumor cells present in the terminal duct lobular units of the breast without light-microscopic evidence of invasion through the basement membrane into the surrounding stroma (Figs. 9.**6** and 9.**7**).

It is widely accepted that LCIS does not represent a precancerous lesion. Instead it appears to be a marker for an increased risk of subsequent invasive breast cancer development at any site in either breast.

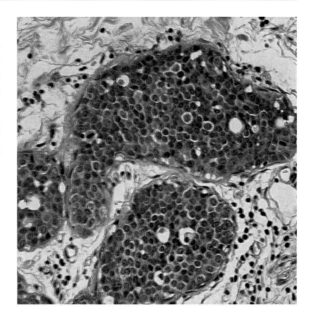

General information

Incidence:	Approximately 20% of all noninvasive breast cancers.
Age peak:	40–50 years (often premenopausal).
Multicentricity:	~50%.
Bilaterality:	~30%.
Risk of malignant transformation:	10–20%.

Findings

Clinical:	Often occult. Palpable mass in ~10% of cases.
Mammography:	No characteristic Findings
Ultrasonography:	Usually no characteristic Findings

Clinical significance

LCIS is usually an incidental microscopic finding in breast tissue removed for another reason without a correlating characteristic clinical or radiographic finding.

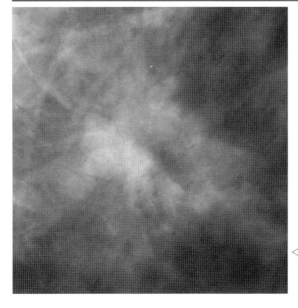

◁ Fig. 9.**6** **LCIS.**
Mammography shows ill-defined hyperdensity within parenchyma.
Histology: LCIS.

Fig. 9.**7a–d   Extensive LCIS.**
a Normal T1-weighted precontrast examination.
b Subtraction image shows oval, partially ill-defined area with inhomogeneous contrast enhancement.
c Signal intensity curves: Some areas show strong, others moderate initial contrast enhancement with continuous postinitial increase or plateau.
d Documentation of lesion after MR localization (LCIS designated by arrows).
Histology: Lobular carcinoma in situ (<2 cm).

MR mammography: LCIS

T1-weighted sequence (precontrast)
Isointense signal behavior in comparison to surrounding breast parenchyma. No specific changes indicating the presence of a LCIS lesion.

T1-weighted sequence (contrast-enhanced)
Approximately one-third of the cases in our own patient collective show an ill-defined contrast-enhancing area with unspecific signal intensity curve. In most cases, however, there is no finding prospectively indicating the presence of malignancy. No detailed reports are found in the current literature.

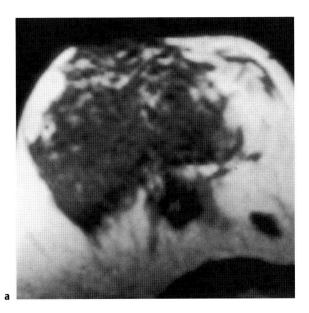

a

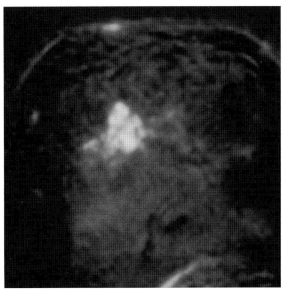

b

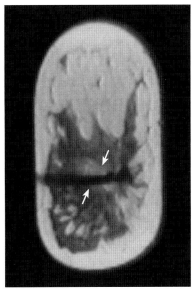

c

d

Invasive Tumor Forms

Invasive Ductal Carcinoma

(Synonyms: invasive duct carcinoma; NOS = not otherwise specified)

Invasive ductal carcinoma is defined as the most frequently encountered malignant tumor of the breast not falling into any of the other categories of invasive mammary carcinoma because specific histological differentiation patterns are lacking or partial. The tumor cells initially develop in the terminal ducts, and tumor cells infiltrate the basal membrane in a single place or in several places. Invasive ductal carcinomas possess a strong fibrotic component. In addition, an extensive intraductal component is often present, which can involve an area more than one-fourth of that of the invasive tumor portion. In general, the tumor form can be described as having a spiculated or circumscribed configuration (Figs. 9.**8**–9.**16**).

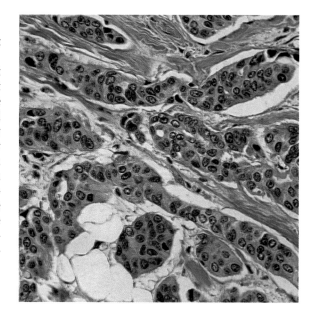

General information	
Grading:	*Histological grade*: well differentiated (GI), intermediate (GII), poorly differentiated (GIII).
Incidence:	Most common form of invasive breast cancer (65–75%).
Age peak:	All ages, peak between 50 and 60 years
Prognosis:	More favorable for well-circumscribed lesions than for spiculated forms. GI better than GII; GII better than GIII.
Multifocality:	15%.
Bilaterality:	5%.

Findings	
Clinical:	Typical criteria of breast cancer: hard, ill-defined mass, often poorly movable and indolent, occasionally skin or nipple retraction (70% of breast cancers are first palpated by the patient!).
Mammography:	Lesion with increased central radiodensity; discrepancy between size in mammography and on palpation. Very variable configuration: spiculated, ill-defined, lobulated, occasionally round or oval. Clustered, pleomorphic microcalcifications in ~30% of cases.
Ultrasonography:	Usually ill-defined, hypoechoic lesion with hyperechoic margins. Central or peripheral posterior acoustic shadowing.

Clinical significance

Most common morphologically variable malignant breast tumor.

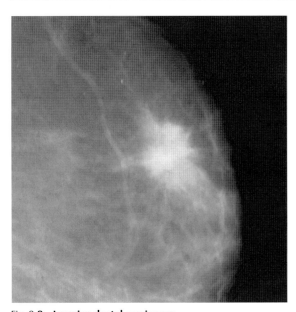

Fig. 9.**8** **Invasive ductal carcinoma.**
Spiculated, high-density lesion in mammography.

MR mammography: Invasive ductal carcinoma

T1-weighted sequence (precontrast)
Isointense signal behavior in comparison to surrounding breast parenchyma and therefore no specific changes allowing demarcation of lesion when located within parenchyma. When the lesion is surrounded by adipose tissue it is seen as a hypointense, occasionally round or ovoid, more often spiculated lesion with ill-defined borders. The spatial resolution of MR mammography does not allow the depiction of pleomorphic microcalcifications.

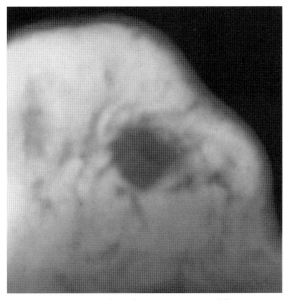

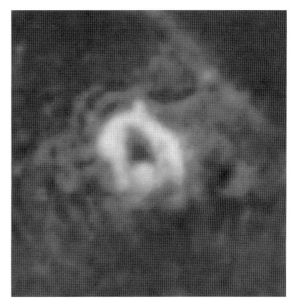

Fig. 9.**9a, b** **Invasive ductal carcinoma; round form.**
a T1-weighted precontrast image shows round lesion within surrounding intramammary adipose tissue.

b Lesion displays typical ring enhancement in subtraction image.

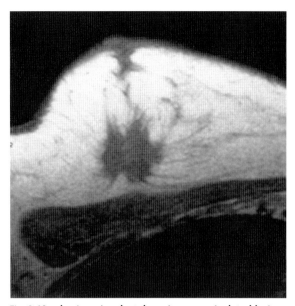

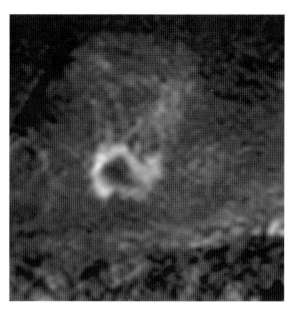

Fig. 9.**10 a, b   Invasive ductal carcinoma; spiculated lesion.**
a T1-weighted precontrast image shows spiculated lesion within surrounding intramammary adipose tissue.

b Lesion displays typical ring enhancement with ill-defined borders in subtraction image.

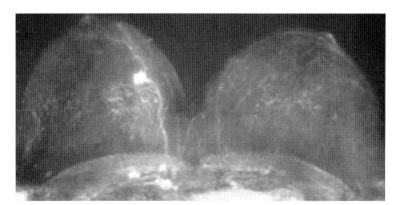

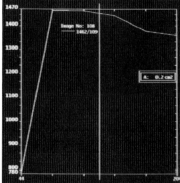

Fig. 9.**11 a, b   Invasive ductal carcinoma.**
a Ill-defined, hypervascularized lesion in the medial portion of the right breast showing CM in draining vein. Rare case with depiction of lymph node metastasis in the right internal mammary lymph node chain. No overlap by cardiac artifacts (MIP image).

b Representative signal intensity curve analysis showing moderate initial contrast enhancement with postinitial plateau. Histology: Invasive ductal carcinoma with lymph node metastasis.

MR mammography: Invasive ductal carcinoma

T2-weighted sequence
In comparison to breast parenchyma the lesion shows similar or slightly lower signal intensity. Occasional exhibition of a peritumoral hyperintense edematous zone.

T1-weighted sequence (contrast-enhanced)
Almost without exception these lesions are round, ovoid, or spiculated and display a contrast enhancement behavior typical of malignancy. Lesion borders are often ill-defined. Ring-enhancement is seen in up to 50% of cases, occasionally with centripetal contrast kinetics. In the signal analysis ~35% of lesions display a moderate and ~60% a strong initial contrast enhancement. Very few lesions display only slight initial contrast enhancement (~5%). In the postinitial phase a plateau is seen most frequently; less frequently one finds a wash-out phenomenon. A continuous signal increase in the postinitial phase rare. As a possible side finding one may see dilated tumor veins.

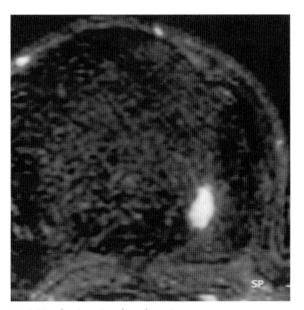

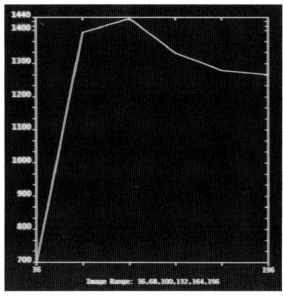

Fig. 9.**12 a, b   Invasive ductal carcinoma.**
a Subtraction image shows oval, ill-defined lesion.

b Signal analysis shows strong initial contrast enhancement with postinitial "wash-out".
Histology: Invasive ductal carcinoma, pT1 GII.

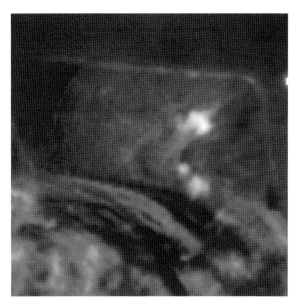

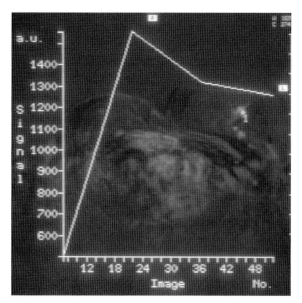

Fig. 9.13 a, b   Invasive ductal carcinoma.

a Subtraction image shows several hypervascularized, ill-defined lesions in the left breast.

b Signal analysis shows strong initial contrast enhancement with postinitial "wash-out".
Histology: Multifocal, invasive ductal carcinoma.

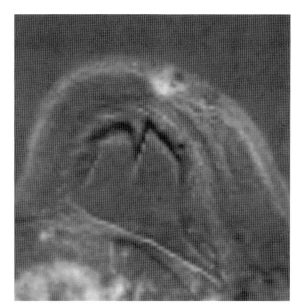

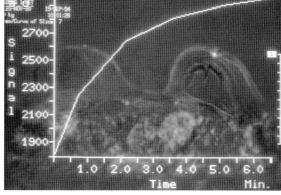

Fig. 9.14 a, b   Invasive ductal carcinoma in postoperative scar.

a Subtraction image shows retroareolar area with increased contrast enhancement.
Note motion artifacts.

b Signal analysis shows atypical signal intensity curve with slight initial contrast enhancement and continuous postinitial signal increase.
Histology: Invasive ductal carcinoma in a postoperative scar.

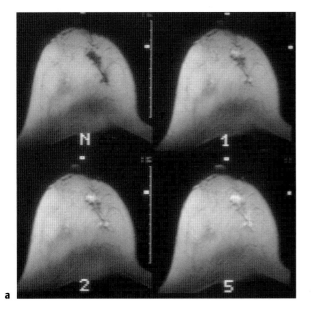

a

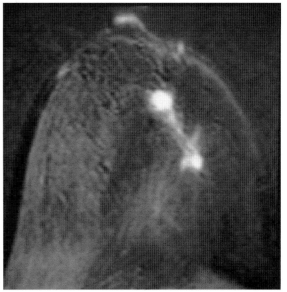

b

Fig. 9.**15 a–c   Multifocal, invasive ductal carcinoma.**
a   Dynamic MR mammography shows two ill-defined, spiculated lesions connected by a tumor bridge.
b   Subtraction image.
c   Signal analysis shows unspecific behavior with moderate initial contrast enhancement and postinitial plateau.
Histology: Multifocal, invasive ductal carcinoma.

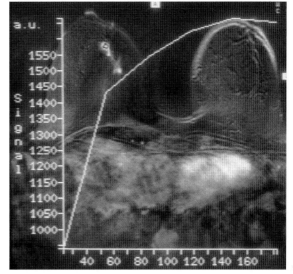

c

Fig. 9.**16 a, b   Invasive ductal carcinoma.**
a   Centrally located, hypervascularized, ill-defined tumor with
spiculations radiating to the periphery.
b   Signal analysis shows strong initial contrast enhancement
with postinitial plateau.
Histology: Invasive ductal carcinoma (pT1) with extensive intraductal component.   ▽

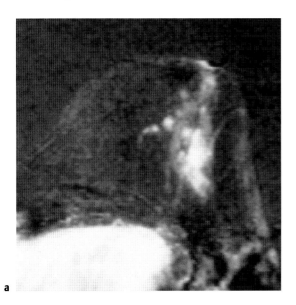

a

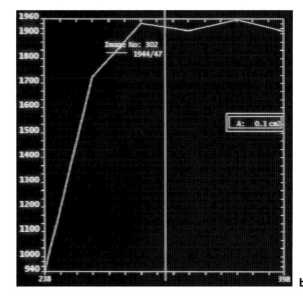

b

Results of Literature Survey

With respect to MR mammography, invasive ductal carcinoma is the best-studied of all breast cancers. Reports from various groups on the sensitivity of this method are in general agreement and document values between 95% and 98%. The few reports of lower sensitivity are predominantly due to technical or methodological shortcomings. Thus, MRI of the breast is currently the most sensitive method in the detection of invasive breast cancer (Table 9.**2**).

Reports of the detection of invasive breast cancer solely in MR mammography substantiate the value of this diagnostic method. The reports from various groups are based primarily on the performance of MR mammography in the preoperative setting for patients with a suspicious breast lesion detected by other imaging techniques. Table 9.**3** presents a summary of the respective study results.

Table 9.**2** Invasive Ductal Carcinoma: Sensitivity of MR Mammography

Authors (year)	No. of Patients	Sensitivity
Boné et al. (1996)	130	100%
Fischer et al. (1999)	233	97%[1]
Gilles et al. (1994)	29	97%
Harms et al. (1993)	46	96%[2]
Kaiser (1993)	130	99%[3]
Klengel et al. (1994)	10	100%[4]
Orel et al. (1995)	43	100%
Stomper et al. (1995)	22	100%

[1] 2× strong enhancement in surrounding tissue, 1× technical mistake, 3× delayed tumor enhancement.
[2] Two carcinomas misinterpreted as physiological mamillary enhancement.
[3] One carcinoma outside the measurement field, 1× overlap of phase-encoding gradient artifact.
[4] 0.5 T examination system.

Table 9.**3** Significance of MRI in the Detection of Invasive Breast Cancer

Authors (year)	No. of Patients	Indication	No. of Carcinomas Detected Solely in MRI[1]
Boetes et al. (1995)	60	Preoperative	9
Fischer et al. (1999)	463	Preoperative	35
Harms et al. (1993)	30	Preoperative	11
Heywang-Köbrunner (1993)	169	Problem cases	14
Krämer et al. (1998)	46	Preoperative	9
Oellinger et al. (1993)	33	Preoperative	8
Orel et al. (1995)	167	Preoperative	22
Rieber et al. (1997)	34	Preoperative	5
Schorn et al. (1999)	14	Search for unknown primary	6

[1] All tumors invasive, predominantly ductal forms.

Invasive Lobular Carcinoma

(Synonym: infiltrating lobular carcinoma)

Invasive lobular carcinoma (Figs. 9.**17** and 9.**20**) is characterized histologically by a desmoplastic stromal reaction, the linear arrangement of tumor cells, a tendency to grow circumferentially around ducts and lobules (so-called "Indian-file" and "targetoid" growth patterns), and the presence of small tumor cells. In some tumors so-called "signet ring cells" (tumor cells with central mucoid globules) are found in addition to the small monomorphic cells. Diffuse and nodular growth patterns are differentiated (Figs. 9.**18** and 9.**19**).

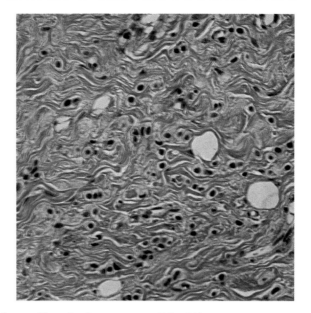

General information

Incidence:	Second most common form of invasive breast cancer (10–15%).
Age peak:	All ages; peak between 40 and 60 years
Multifocality:	~30%.
Prognosis:	Comparatively bad (due to late diagnosis). Occasionally unusual patterns of metastatic spread (e.g., intra-abdominal, intrapelvic, retroperitoneal).
Multifocality	Twice that of ductal carcinoma (30%).
Bilaterality:	Twice that of ductal carcinoma (10%).

Findings

Clinical:	Variable from occult to large, palpable mass.
Mammography:	*Diffuse* type: architectural distortion, localized changes in density, or structural irregularities. Rarely tumor-associated microcalcifications.
	Nodular type: often focal, ill-defined hyperdensity displaying characteristic signs of malignancy.
Ultrasonography:	*Diffuse* type: often diffuse hypoechoic changes.
	Nodular type: focal lesions with typical characteristics of malignancy.

Clinical significance

Invasive lobular carcinoma has the lowest detection rate of carcinomas in all breast imaging techniques, and is therefore occasionally first diagnosed at a late stage.

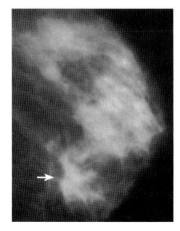

Fig. 9.**17**   **Invasive lobular carcinoma.**
Spiculated, isodense mass in the caudal portion of the left breast.

MR mammography: Invasive lobular carcinoma

T1-weighted sequence (precontrast)
Isointense signal behavior in comparison to surrounding breast parenchyma, therefore no specific changes allowing demarcation of the lesion when located within parenchyma. When it is surrounded by adipose tissue, the lesion is seen as hypointense round or ill-defined (especially of the nodular type). This precontrast examination is most often without conspicuous findings.

T2-weighted sequence
The lesion shows signal intensity similar to or slightly lower than that of breast parenchyma. Occasionally a peritumoral hyperintense edematous zone is exhibited.

T1-weighted sequence (contrast-enhanced)
Usually these lesions are round, irregular, or spiculated and display a contrast enhancement typical of malignancy. Lesion borders are often ill-defined. The nodular type shows a ring-enhancement in up to 50% of cases. The signal analysis shows a moderate to strong initial contrast enhancement. Occasional lesions display only slight initial contrast enhancement. In the postinitial phase, a plateau is seen most frequently; less frequently one finds a wash-out phenomenon. A continuous signal increase in the postinitial phase is possible, however. The detection rate of invasive lobular carcinomas in MR mammography is lower than that of invasive ductal carcinomas (Table 9.**4**).

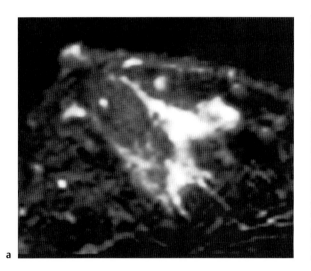

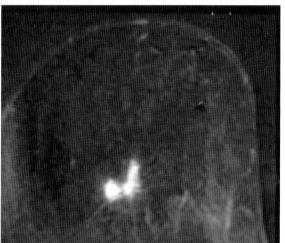

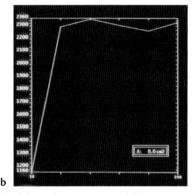

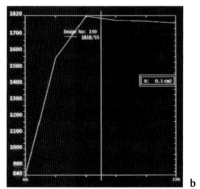

Fig. 9.**18 a, b Invasive lobular breast cancer, diffuse type.**
a Subtraction image shows diffuse contrast enhancement in central portions of the breast with dendritic lines radiating toward the periphery.
b Signal analysis shows strong initial contrast enhancement with postinitial plateau.
Histology (large-core biopsy): Invasive lobular carcinoma GII.

Fig. 9.**19 a, b Invasive lobular breast cancer, nodular type.**
a Subtraction image shows adjacent round and ovoid tumors with ill-defined borders in central portion of left breast.
b Signal analysis shows strong initial contrast enhancement with postinitial plateau.
Histology: Invasive lobular carcinoma pT2 GII.

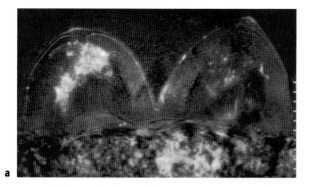
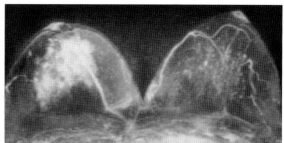
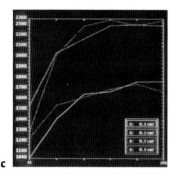
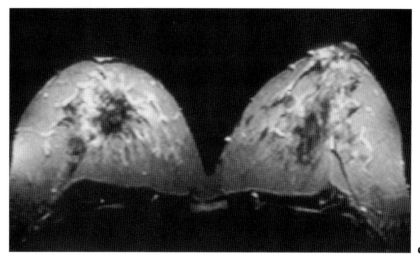

Fig. 9.**20 a–d   Invasive lobular carcinoma.**
a Single slice subtraction image shows extensive area with contrast enhancement.
b Presentation of entire extent of tumor in MIP technique.
c Varying signal intensity curves, some demonstrating characteristics of malignancy.

d T2-weighted examination shows hypointense tumor center. Peritumoral edema.
Histology (large-core biopsy before neoadjuvant therapy): Invasive lobular carcinoma.

Results of Literature Survey

Invasive lobular carcinoma is a great challenge for all breast imaging techniques. Diffuse forms of this type of breast cancer in particular are occasionally difficult to detect. Reports in the medical literature substantiate the limited sensitivity of MR mammography in the detection of this form of tumor. Despite this, MR mammography has proven itself to be superior to other breast imaging techniques in the detection and in the preoperative assessment and documentation of tumor dimensions (Table 9.**4**).

Table 9.**4**   Invasive Lobular Carcinoma: Sensitivity of MR Mammography

Authors (year)	Number	Criterion	Sensitivity of MRI
Fischer et al. (1999)	24	Detection	92 %[1]
Rodenko et al. (1996)	20	Extent	100 %
		Morphology	91 %
Sittek et al.(1998)	23	Detection	83 %[2]

[1] One false-negative case with slight contrast enhancement; one false-negative case due to diffuse enhancement of surrounding parenchyma.
[2] Two false-negative cases without contrast enhancement; two false-negative cases due to diffuse enhancement of surrounding parenchyma.

Medullary Carcinoma

The histopathological features that define the *typical form of medullary carcinoma* are a tendency for tumor cells to grow in broad sheets without distinct cell borders (syncytial pattern), high nuclear grade (pleomorphic nuclei with prominent nucleoli, usually accompanied by a high mitotic rate), circumscribed tumor margins, and an intense lymphoplasmacytic reaction around and within the tumor. Carcinomas that have most, but not all, of these microscopic features are referred to as *atypical medullary carcinomas*. The median size of medullary carcinomas is 2–3 cm. Lesions larger than 5 cm tend to show central tumor necrosis and calcification (Figs. 9.**21**–9.**23**).

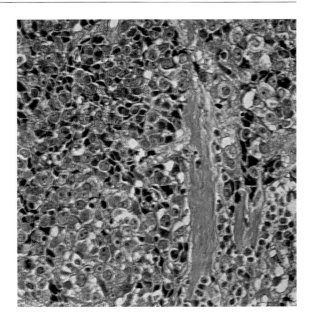

─ General information

Incidence:	Rare. Less that 10% of all mammary carcinomas. Often associated with *BRCA* gene.
Age peak:	All ages; usually under 50 years
Prognosis:	*Typical form*: more favorable than that of invasive ductal carcinoma.
	Atypical form: identical with that of invasive ductal carcinoma.

─ Findings

Clinical:	Well-circumscribed tumor.
Mammography:	Well-circumscribed, round or lobulated mass.
	Occasionally partially ill-defined borders due to lymphocytic infiltrates.
Ultrasonography:	Well-circumscribed, rounded hypoechoic lesion.

─ Clinical significance

Medullary carcinoma has a special significance within the group of malignant mammary tumors because its typical form is occasionally difficult to differentiate from solid benign tumors of the breast (e.g., fibroadenoma).

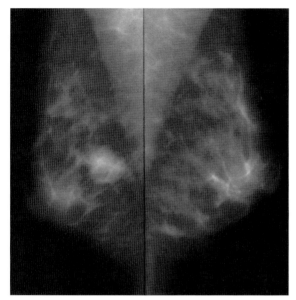

Fig. 9.21 Medullary carcinoma of the breast.
Mammography shows a well-circumscribed round mass in the central portion of the right breast.

 MR mammography: Medullary carcinoma

T1-weighted sequence (precontrast)
Well-circumscribed, hypointense lesion, difficult to detect when located within parenchyma.

T2-weighted sequence
In comparison to breast parenchyma, lesion shows similar or slightly lower signal intensity. Occasional exhibition of peritumoral hyperintense edematous zone.

T1-weighted sequence (contrast-enhanced)
Round or ovoid lesion displaying a contrast enhancement pattern typical of malignancy. Occasional demonstration of ring-enhancement. Signal analysis usually shows moderate to strong initial contrast enhancement. Rare lesions display only slight initial contrast enhancement. In the postinitial phase a plateau is most frequently seen; less frequently one finds a wash-out phenomenon. A continuous signal increase in the postinitial phase is very rare.

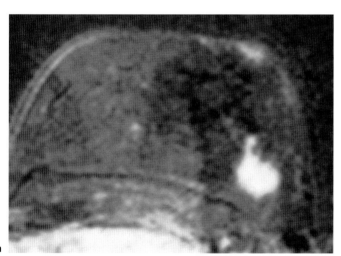

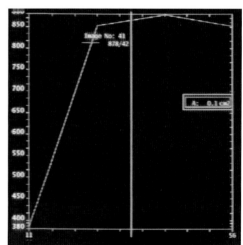

Fig. 9.22 a, b Medullary carcinoma.
a Subtraction image shows round lesion with small satellite-like extension.

b Signal analysis shows strong initial contrast enhancement with postinitial plateau.
Histology: Medullary carcinoma pT2 GII.

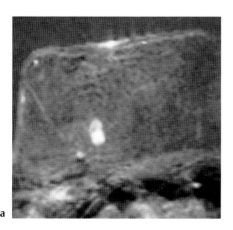

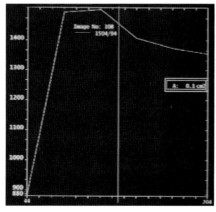

Fig. 9.23 a, b Medullary carcinoma.
a Subtraction image shows an oval lesion with partially ill-defined margins.
b Signal analysis shows moderate initial contrast enhancement with postinitial wash-out phenomenon.
Histology: Medullary carcinoma pT1 GII.

Mucinous Carcinoma

The histopathological characteristic that defines the *typical form of mucinous carcinoma* is the accumulation of abundant extracellular mucinous secretion around islandlike clusters of tumor cells. Calcifications are rarely found. The *atypical or mixed form of mucinous carcinoma* is regarded as a variant of ductal or otherwise differentiated carcinoma with a low proportion of mucinous secretion (25–50% of tumor volume).

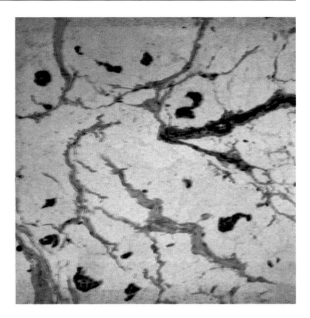

General information

Incidence:	Rare. Approximately 1–4% of all mammary carcinomas.
Age peak:	All ages; proportionately more older women.
Prognosis:	*Typical form*: favorable prognosis.
	Atypical form: identical with that of invasive ductal carcinoma.

Findings

Clinical:	Well-circumscribed tumor.
Mammography:	Well-circumscribed, round or lobulated mass (Fig. 9.**24**).
	Occasionally partially ill-defined borders.
	Rarely tumor-associated microcalcifications
Ultrasonography:	Well-circumscribed, often hyperechoic, less frequently hypoechoic lesion.

Clinical significance

Depending upon the extent of the mucinous component, mucinous carcinomas have a favorable prognosis in comparison to other mammary carcinomas.

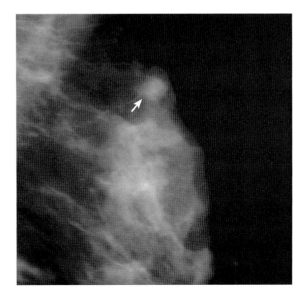

Fig. 9.**24** **Mucinous carcinoma of the breast.**
Mammography shows a well-circumscribed, round lesion with partially ill-defined margins (arrow) in the left breast.

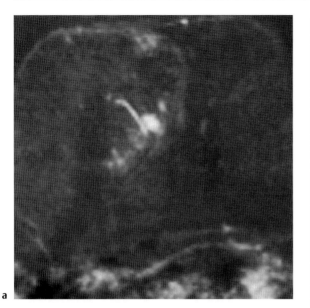

a

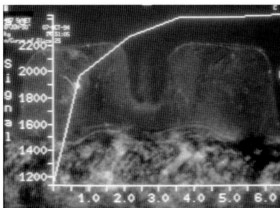

b

 MR mammography: Mucinous carcinoma

T1-weighted sequence (precontrast)
Well-circumscribed, hypointense lesion, difficult to detect when located within parenchyma.

T2-weighted sequence
In comparison to breast parenchyma, lesion typically shows similar or slightly lower signal intensity.

T1-weighted sequence (contrast-enhanced)
Round or ovoid, well-circumscribed lesion displaying contrast enhancement. Rare demonstration of ring-enhancement. Signal analysis frequently shows very strong initial contrast enhancement (>200% of precontrast values). Occasionally only moderate initial contrast enhancement. Rare lesions display only slight initial contrast enhancement. In the postinitial phase a plateau is seen most frequently; less frequently one finds a wash-out phenomenon. A continuous signal increase in the postinitial phase is very rare.
Cave: Cases of mucinous carcinomas without contrast enhancement do exist (Fig. 9.**26**).

Fig. 9.**25 a, b   Mucinous carcinoma.**
a   Subtraction image shows oval lesion with adjacent vein.
b   Signal analysis shows moderate initial contrast enhancement with postinitial plateau.
Histology: Mucinous carcinoma.

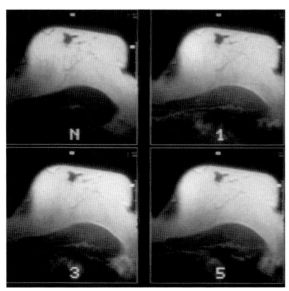

a

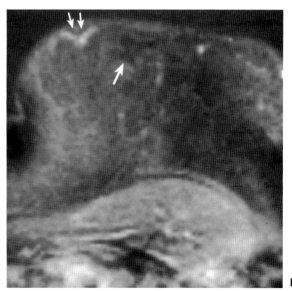

b

Fig. 9.**26 a, b   Mucinous carcinoma. MR mammographic pitfall.**
a   Dynamic measurements demonstrate lesion without contrast enhancement (1, 3, 5 minutes post-CM).

b   Subtraction image. Lack of contrast enhancement within carcinoma (arrow) (mammography Fig. 9.**24**). Normal contrast enhancement in intramammary vein (double arrows).
Histology: Mucinous carcinoma.

Invasive Papillary Carcinoma

The term *invasive papillary carcinoma* is used to describe carcinomas that have a frond-forming microscopic growth pattern. In addition, these lesions often have a cystic component (Figs. 9.**27**–9.**29**). **Intraductal papillary carcinomas** and **noninvasive intracystic papillary carcinomas** must be differentiated from invasive papillary carcinomas.

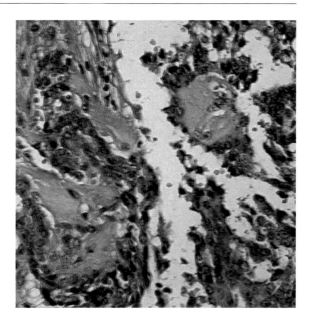

General information

Incidence:	Rare. ApproxImately 2% of all mammary carcinomas.
Age peak:	50–60 years.
Prognosis:	Identical with that of invasive ductal carcinoma.

Findings

Clinical:	Circumscribed, subareolar tumor, bloody nipple discharge, nipple retraction.
Mammography:	Ill-defined, often lobulated lesion.
	Asymmetric density in retroareolar region.
	Rarely tumor-associated microcalcifications
Ultrasonography:	Ill-defined, hypoechoic or anechoic lesion with hyperechoic wall. Central or peripheral posterior shadowing.

Clinical significance

The possible presence of an invasive papillary carcinoma must be considered if the tumor does not respect the borders of the cyst wall.

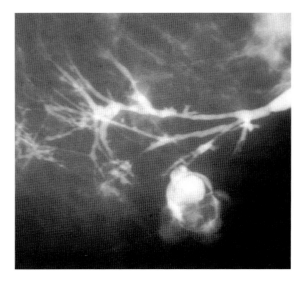

Fig. 9.**27** **Invasive papillary carcinoma.**
Galactography shows incomplete filling of a solitary sacculary duct dilatation in an otherwise normal duct system.
Histology: Invasive papillary carcinoma pT1 GII.

MR mammography: Invasive papillary carcinoma

T1-weighted sequence (precontrast)
Usually well-circumscribed, hypointense lesion in retroareolar region of the breast.

T2-weighted sequence
Occasional disruption of wall contours of a signal-intense cyst by a well-circumscribed lesion with intermediary signal intensity.

T1-weighted sequence (contrast-enhanced)
Usually round or ovoid, well-circumscribed lesion displaying prominent contrast enhancement. Most often signal analysis shows strong initial contrast enhancement with postinitial plateau or wash-out. Possible ring enhancement.

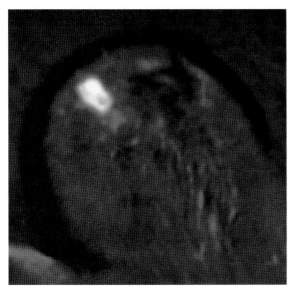

Fig. 9.**28 a, b   Invasive papillary carcinoma** (see galactography in Fig. 9.**27**).
a Subtraction image shows an oval, hypervascularized tumor with peripheral accentuation of contrast enhancement in the lower medial portion of the right breast.

b Signal analysis shows almost 100% initial contrast enhancement with postinitial plateau.
Histology: Invasive papillary carcinoma pT1 GII.

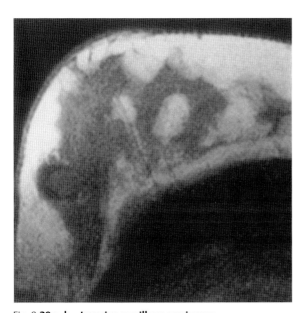

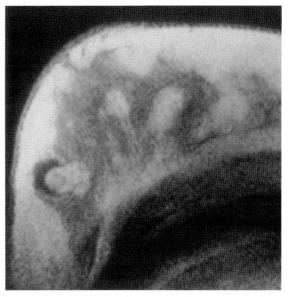

Fig. 9.**29 a, b   Invasive papillary carcinoma.**
a T1-weighted GE sequence shows solid lesion within a cystic lesion.

b Prominent contrast enhancement of intracystic and extracystic tumor portions.
Histology: Invasive papillary carcinoma pT1 GII.

Tubular Carcinoma

The typical *tubular carcinoma* is characterized by a pro-liferation of well-differentiated, often angular or branching tubular neoplastic elements resembling normal breast ductules. These are lined by a single layer of cuboid epithelium. At least 75% of the tumor must have a tubular growth pattern to qualify for this diagnosis. Tubular carcinoma is accompanied by a strong fibrotic and myxoid component. Tumor margins are often stellate (Figs. 9.**30**–9.**32**). Microcalcifications are found in ~50% of cases. Tumors with tubular elements constituting less than 75% are referred to as *mixed tubular carcinomas*.

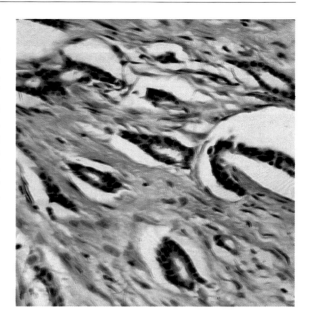

── General information

Incidence:	Rare. Less than 2% of all mammary carcinomas.
Age peak:	All ages; peak between 50 and 60 years
Prognosis:	Favorable in comparison with that of invasive ductal carcinoma.

── Findings

Clinical:	Palpable suspicious tumor.
Mammography:	Ill-defined, often stellate lesion with prominent spiculae. Occasional architectural distortion. Microcalcifications in >50% of cases.
Ultrasonography:	Ill-defined, hypoechoic lesion with posterior acoustic extinction.

── Clinical significance

Tubular carcinomas often arise from benign proliferative lesions called radial scars. It has been suggested that, as they enlarge, tubular carcinomas are converted into ordinary invasive duct carcinomas.

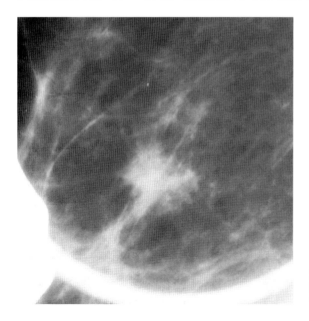

Fig. 9.**30**   **Tubular carcinoma.**
Mammography shows stellate hyperdensity (spot compression view).

MR mammography: Tubular carcinoma

T1-weighted sequence (precontrast)
Stellate, hypointense lesion that is difficult to detect when located within parenchyma. When located within adipose tissue, the lesion demonstrates suspicious characteristics.

T2-weighted sequence
In comparison to breast parenchyma, the lesion shows similar or slightly lower signal intensity. Occasional exhibition of peritumoral hyperintense edematous zone.

T1-weighted sequence (contrast-enhanced)
Stellate lesion displaying a contrast enhancement pattern typical of malignancy. Rare demonstration of ring-enhancement. Signal analysis usually shows moderate to strong initial contrast enhancement. Rare lesions display only slight initial contrast enhancement. In the postinitial phase a plateau is seen most frequently; less frequently one finds a wash-out phenomenon. A continuous signal increase in the postinitial phase is very rare.

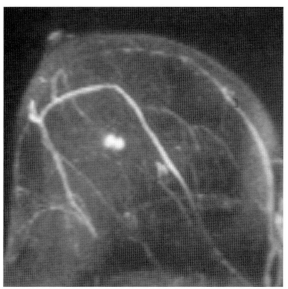
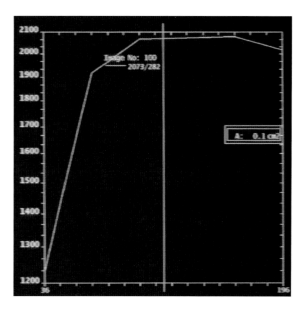

Fig. 9.**31 a, b Tubular carcinoma.**
a Subtraction image shows two adjacent, hypervascularized lesions.

b Signal analysis shows moderate initial contrast enhancement with postinitial plateau.
Histology: Tubular carcinoma pT1 GII.

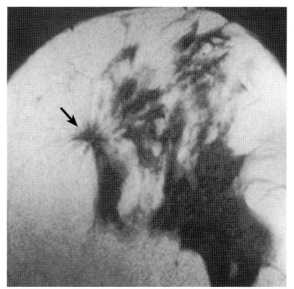
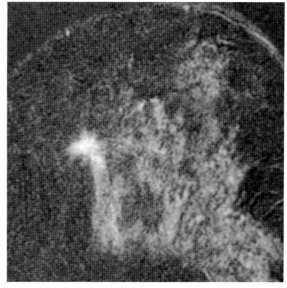

Fig. 9.**32 a, b Tubular carcinoma.**
a T1-weighted image shows a stellate lesion in the central portion of the right breast (arrow).

b In the subtraction image this lesion shows a stronger contrast enhancement than the surrounding parenchyma.
Histology: Tubular carcinoma pT1 GII.

Other Tumor Forms

Inflammatory Carcinoma

Inflammatory carcinoma does not constitute a histological type but rather a clinical entity (Figs. 9.**33**–9.**35**). Microscopically there is a diffuse infiltration of the skin and mammary tissue, usually by a poorly differentiated infiltrating duct carcinoma. The striking clinical manifestation of inflammatory carcinoma is erythema and edema usually involving more than one-third of the breast skin. In ~80% of cases one finds tumor cells within the dilated dermal lymphatic channels.

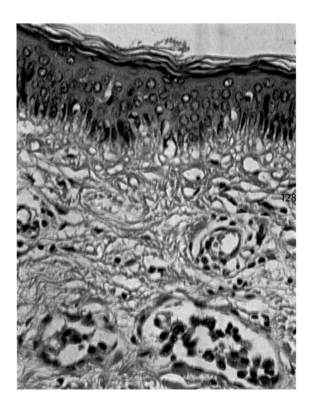

General information

Incidence:	Rare (1–2% of all mammary carcinomas).
Age peak:	40–60 years.
Bilaterality:	Relatively high (reports up to 30%).
Prognosis:	Very bad. Most aggressive form of all mammary carcinomas.

Findings

Clinical (method of choice):	Erythema. Edema. Hyperthermia. Pain. Diffusely increased firmness. Enlarged skin pores, peau d'orange, cancer en cuirass, tumor fixation. Often enlarged axillary lymph nodes (due to metastases).
Mammography:	Skin thickening. Increased density of parenchyma (note asymmetry!). Occasionally diffuse pleomorphic microcalcifications. Circumscribed mass visible in only one-third of cases.
Ultrasonography:	Skin thickening, interstitial fluid collections (note asymmetry!).

Clinical significance

Inflammatory carcinoma is very difficult to distinguish from nonpuerperal mastitis clinically, as well as with breast imaging techniques. Biopsy of the skin is, therefore, one of the first diagnostic procedures performed to make this distinction.

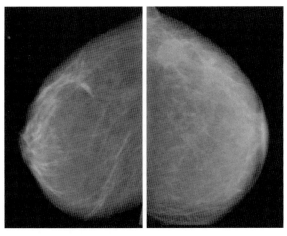

Fig. 9.33 Inflammatory breast carcinoma.
Mammography shows unilateral diffusely increased density of parenchyma, reticular patterning of subcutaneous area, and skin thickening of the left breast. Note the obvious tumor in the upper outer quadrant.

MR mammography: Inflammatory carcinoma

T1-weighted sequence (precontrast)
Skin thickening is often the only feature suggestive of malignancy (differential diagnosis: irradiated breast, nonpuerperal mastitis).

T2-weighted sequence
Diffuse increase in signal intensity of affected breast in comparison with contralateral breast. Skin thickening.

T1-weighted sequence (contrast-enhanced)
Increased contrast enhancement of thickened skin and parenchymal structures infiltrated by tumor. Occasionally signal analysis does not show typical characteristics of malignancy (reports exist of slight to moderate initial contrast enhancement with continual postinitial signal increase). Occasional documentation of primary tumorous lesion.
Cave: There are case reports of no or slight contrast enhancement when clinical symptoms are absent or mild in spite of the presence of cutaneous lymphatic tumor emboli (*occult inflammatory carcinoma*). The apparent reason is the predominant diffuse spread of tumor cells through the lymphatic septa in the absence of tumor angiogenesis.

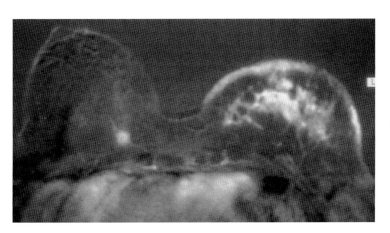

Fig. 9.34 Inflammatory breast carcinoma.
Single slice subtraction image shows skin thickening with increased enhancement, as well as prominent enhancement of central portions of the left breast. Simultaneous growth of contralateral breast cancer in the medial portion of the right breast. Histological confirmation of both diagnoses.

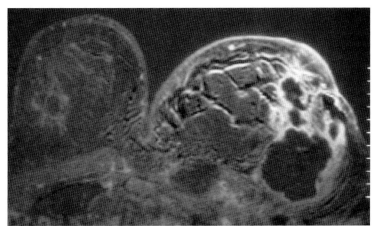

Fig. 9.35 Inflammatory breast carcinoma.
Single slice subtraction image shows moderate skin thickening and prominent increase of enhancement in cutaneous and intramammary structures. Demarcation of extensive necrosis with formation of tumor cavities. Tumor infiltration of the pectoralis muscle.
Diagnosis confirmed histologically.

Paget Disease of the Nipple

Paget disease should be viewed as a ductal carcinoma in situ involving the nipple (Figs. 9.**36**–9.**39**). Large, ovoid tumor cells, called *Paget cells*, are found singularly or in aggregates within the epidermis of the nipple and may spread to the surrounding skin areas. In advanced stages, ulcerations but not infiltration of the corium can be seen.

Paget disease of the nipple is typically associated with DCIS (60%) or invasive carcinoma (30%) of the breast.

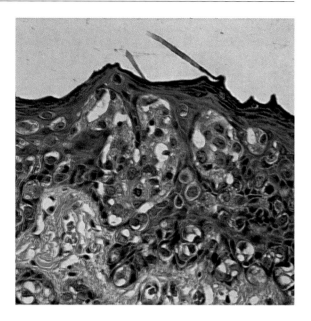

General information

Incidence:	Rare. Approximately 2% of all mammary carcinomas.
Age peak:	All ages; peak between 40 and 60 years.
Prognosis	Usually favorable (depending on intramammary manifestation).

Findings

Clinical	Nonhealing eczematoid changes of the nipple and/or areola.
(method of choice):	Palpable mass in ~60% of cases.
Mammography:	Occasional flattening or thickening of nipple region; retromamillary density. Retromamillary microcalcifications in ~50% of cases.
Ultrasonography:	Rare demonstration of diagnostically relevant findings.

Clinical significance

The primary differential diagnoses of Paget disease are dermatological diseases. Confirmation of Paget disease of the nipple may be achieved by exfoliative cytology or skin biopsy.

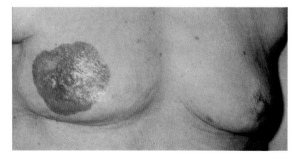

Fig. 9.36   Paget disease of the nipple.
Typical eczematoid changes in the right nipple and surrounding skin. Asymmetric flattening of the right nipple region.

MR mammography: Paget disease of the nipple

T1-weighted sequence (precontrast)
Possible flattening and/or thickening of mamillary region.

T2-weighted sequence
Rare documentation of asymmetric subareolar hyperintensity.

T1-weighted sequence (contrast-enhanced)
Variable findings ranging from no contrast enhancement in the mamillary region, to findings typical of malignancy with strong initial contrast enhancement and postinitial plateau or wash-out phenomenon. Occasionally MR mammography provides additional diagnostic information pertaining to the presence and extent of the intramammary tumor (DCIS, invasive carcinoma).

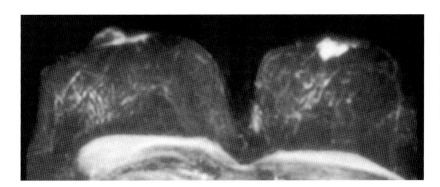

Fig. 9.37 Paget disease of the nipple.
Subtraction image shows a localized enhancing area in the left mamillary and subareolar region. Physiological mamillary and blood vessel enhancement in the right breast.
Diagnosis confirmed histologically.

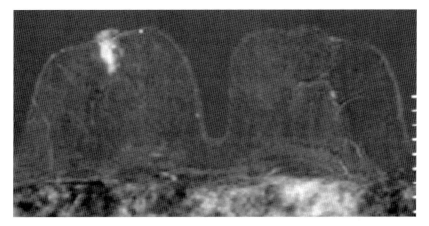

Fig. 9.38 Paget disease of the nipple.
Subtraction image shows contrast enhancement reaching from the areolar region toward the center of the right breast as a sign of involvement of the retromamillary ducts.
Diagnosis confirmed histologically.

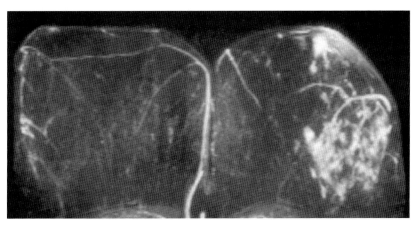

Fig. 9.39 Paget disease of the nipple.
Subtraction image shows increased enhancement in the left mamillary and subareolar region. Additional documentation of extensive intraductal and minimally invasive tumor in the lateral portions of the left breast.
Diagnosis confirmed histologically.

Malignant Phyllodes Tumor

(Synonyms: phyllodes tumor, malignant cystosarcoma phyllodes)

The phyllodes tumor is a distinctive fibroepithelial tumor of the breast without counterpart in any other organ of the body (Figs. 9.**40** and 9.**41**). The malignant form of this tumor is characterized by its high mitotic activity (>5 mitoses/10 HPF), cellular atypia, a dominant stromal component, and a tumor growth pattern that infiltrates the surrounding tissue. The stroma of the tumor shows a predominantly sarcomatous differentiation. In addition, tumors often show signs of hemorrhage and ulcerations.

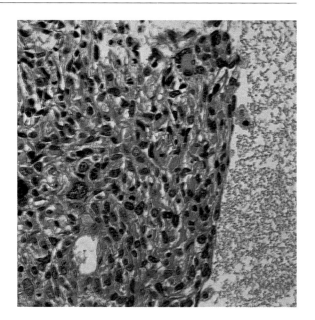

General information

Prognosis:	No reliable data.
Metastatic spread:	Hematogenous in 20% of cases, rarely lymphogenous.
Incidence:	0.2% of all mammary carcinomas.
Age peak:	40–60 years

Findings

Clinical:	Rapidly growing, smooth or tuberous mass, up to 10 cm or more in diameter. Skin changes with large tumors (thinning and/or livid discoloration).
Mammography:	Homogeneous, round, oval, or lobulated tumor (similar to fibroadenoma). Occasional halo sign due to compression of surrounding tissue. Rarely microcalcifications or macrocalcifications.
Ultrasonography:	Smooth-bordered, rounded or lobulated lesion with posterior acoustic enhancement. Cystic inclusions are diagnostically relevant.

Clinical significance

The differential diagnosis between a phyllodes tumor and a fibroadenoma is occasionally difficult. Patient age, rapid growth, and the documentation of cystic inclusions are indicative for a phyllodes tumor.

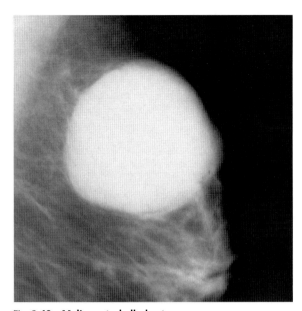

Fig. 9.40 Malignant phyllodes tumor.
Mammography shows a large, well-defined, lobulated mass.

 MR mammography: Malignant phyllodes tumor

T1-weighted sequence (precontrast)

Smooth-bordered, round or lobulated lesion without pseudocapsular demarcation. Signal intensity lower than or equivalent to that of parenchyma. Occasional documentation of rounded inclusions with comparatively hypointense signal as MR equivalent of cystic or necrotic changes.

T2-weighted sequence

Smooth-bordered, round or lobulated lesion with isointense to hyperintense signal in comparison to parenchymal signal intensity. Occasional documentation of rounded inclusions with hyperintense signal as MR equivalent of cystic or necrotic changes.

T1-weighted (contrast-enhanced)

Strong contrast enhancement within solid tumor portions. In the further course of the examination, increasing demarcation of existing cystic or necrotic areas. Initial contrast enhancement is usually 100% or more. Postinitial signal usually shows continuous increase or plateau. When no liquid inclusions are documented, differentiation from a fibroadenoma with a high proportion of stromal tissue is not possible. Differentiation between the benign, malignant, and borderline phyllodes tumors is not possible in MR mammography.

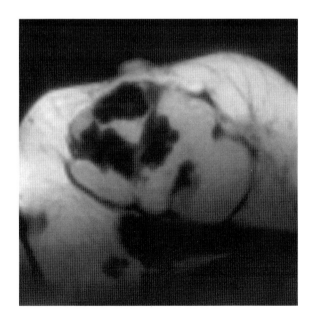 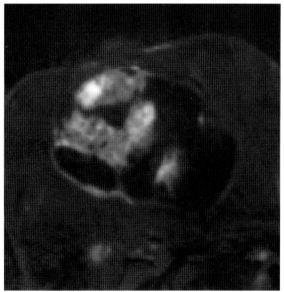

Fig. 9.41 a, b Malignant phyllodes tumor.
a T1-weighted precontrast image shows a lobulated tumor with solid portions (hypointense) and hemorrhagic cystic portions (hyperintense).

b Subtraction image shows inhomogeneous enhancement in solid tumor portions, no enhancement in cystic portions, and partial enhancement of surrounding capsule.
Histology: Malignant phyllodes tumor.

Sarcoma

Breast sarcomas originate in the periductal or perilobular stroma. Consistently with the manifestations of primary malignant mesenchymal tumors in other soft tissues, they represent a heterogeneous histological group. The most common type is the malignant fibrous histiocytoma; less frequent are the angiosarcomas (Figs. 9.**42** and 9.**43**). Rarely, sarcomas may occur following radiotherapy. Fibrosarcomas, malignant fibrous histiocytomas, liposarcomas, leiomyosarcomas, chondrosarcomas, and angiosarcomas in the breast have been reported.

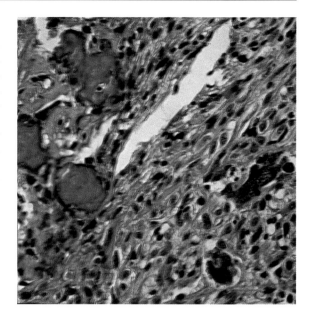

General information

Incidence:	Very rare (<1 % of all malignant breast tumors).
Age peak:	All age groups (mean age 30–40 years).
Prognosis:	Dependent upon histological grade.
Bilaterality:	Very rare.

Findings

Clinical:	Painless, mobile, often fast-growing mass (at time of detection ~4–6 cm). Skin changes with large tumors (stretching, livid discoloration).
Mammography:	High-density, usually well-defined mass, occasionally microlobulated. Presence of endotumoral bony trabecular structures is evidence of osteosarcoma.
Ultrasonography:	Inhomogeneous, hypoechoic structural changes.

Clinical significance

Because breast sarcomas occur very rarely, they are of little clinical significance.

MR mammography: Angiosarcoma

T1-weighted sequence (precontrast)
Usually smooth-bordered lesion without pseudo-capsular demarcation. Signal intensity lower than or equivalent to that of parenchyma. Endotumoral hyperintense regions corresponding to blood clots.

T1-weighted sequence (precontrast + fat saturation)
No signal suppression of endotumoral hyperintense regions.

T2-weighted sequence
Usually smooth-bordered lesion with hyperintense signal in comparison to parenchymal signal intensity. Endotumoral hypointense regions corresponding to blood clots.

T1-weighted (contrast-enhanced)
Smooth-bordered, rounded lesion with inhomogeneous contrast enhancement. Signal analysis shows characteristics typical of malignancy (strong initial contrast enhancement; postinitial plateau or wash-out phenomenon). Endotumoral regions (blood clots) show no contrast enhancement. This appears to be a pathognomonic finding for angiosarcomas (6/6 cases).

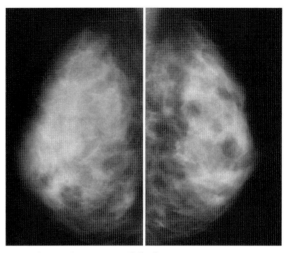
Fig. 9.**42**   **Angiosarcoma of the breast.**

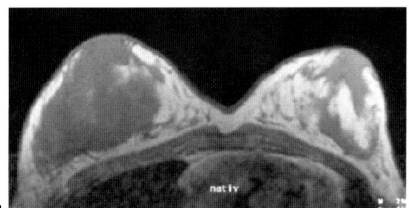

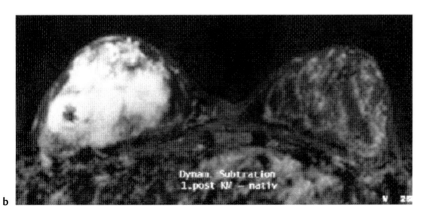

Fig. 9.**43 a, b**   **Angiosarcoma of the breast.**

Metastases to the Breast

Intramammary metastases are a manifestation of a primary malignant tumor most commonly located in the contralateral breast. Other primary tumors are extramammary (e.g., bronchogenic carcinoma, malignant melanoma) or a manifestation of a malignant systemic disease (e.g., lymphomas and leukemia) (Figs. 9.**44**–9.**46**). Rare extramammary primary tumors include plasmocytoma, carcinomas of the kidneys, urinary bladder, ovaries, stomach, and uterus, and intestinal carcinoid tumors. Adenocarcinomas of the colon and rectum are rarely the source of metastatic carcinoma in the breast.

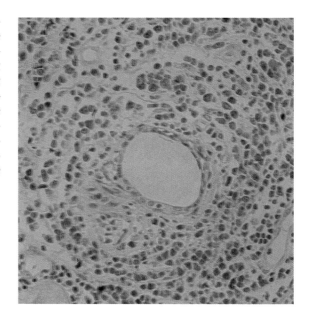

General information

Prognosis:	Usually poor (exceptions: malignant melanomas, lymphomas)
Incidence:	Very rare.
Age peak:	Depends upon primary tumor.
Bilaterality:	Relatively common (reports up to 30%).

Findings

Clinical:	Small intramammary lesions usually occult.
Mammography:	Metastases of solid primary tumors: smooth-bordered, round, homogeneous lesion(s). Metastases of lymphomas or leukemia: diffuse increase of parenchymal density. Rarely microcalcifications or macrocalcifications.
Ultrasonography:	Smooth-bordered, rounded solid lesion(s) with posterior acoustic enhancement. Metastases of lymphomas or leukemia: diffuse increase of parenchymal echogeneity.

Clinical significance

Distinguishing between a primary tumor of the breast and a metastasis to the breast, i.e., hematological or lymphatic systemic disease, is of great importance for therapeutic consequences and prognosis.

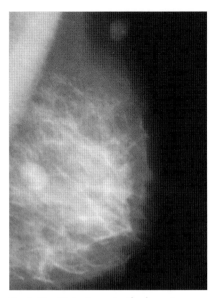

Fig. 9.44 Metastases to the breast.
Mammography shows several well-circumscribed, homogeneous, rounded lesions.

 MR mammography: Metastases to the breast

T1-weighted sequence (precontrast)
Smooth-bordered lesion(s) with signal intensity lower than or equivalent to that of parenchyma and therefore difficult to detect when located within parenchyma. When the lesion is located within adipose tissue, there is clear demarcation and detection is easy. Lymphoma may show skin thickening.

T2-weighted sequence
Smooth-bordered lesion(s) with isointense or slightly hyperintense signal intensity. Diffuse involvement results in higher signal intensity of the corresponding breast (unspecific finding).

T1-weighted (contrast-enhanced)
Smooth-bordered, round or ovoid lesion usually showing strong contrast enhancement. Signal analysis shows characteristics typical of primary breast cancer (strong initial contrast enhancement; postinitial plateau or wash-out phenomenon). Possible ring-enhancement.

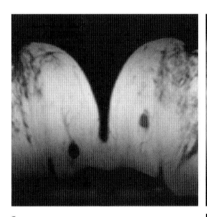
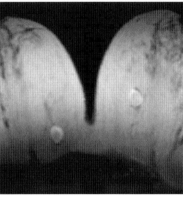
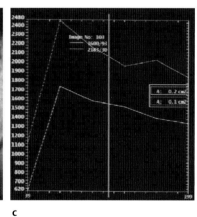

a   b   c

Fig. 9.45 a–c Intramammary metastases of malignant melanoma.

a T1-weighted precontrast image shows oval, hypointense lesions in both breasts.
b Lesions show ring-enhancement in T1-weighted postcontrast image.

c Signal analysis shows strong initial contrast enhancement with postinitial "wash-out".
Cytological confirmation of diagnosis.

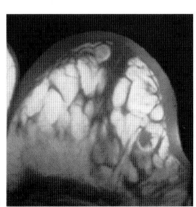
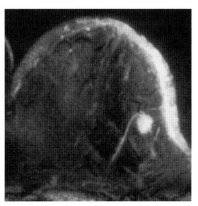

a   b

Fig. 9.46 a, b Manifestation of Hodgkin's lymphoma in the breast.
a T1-weighted precontrast image shows skin thickening.
b T1-weighted postcontrast image shows partial contrast enhancement of the skin (diagnosis confirmed histologically). Additional detection of a hypervascularized, ill-defined lesion in the lateral portion of the breast (cytologically confirmed manifestation of Hodgkin lymphoma).

10   MR Mammography in Men

Gynecomastia

The term *gynecomastia* goes back to Galen (ca. 129–200). It describes a benign, usually reversible, unilateral or bilateral enlargement of the male breast (Fig. 10.**1**). Gynecomastia is due to an increase in breast stroma and, to a lesser extent, ductal proliferation. It is classified into several different categories and may be a normal physiological phenomenon or a pathological finding associated with an underlying disease.

Neonatal Gynecomastia, Pubertal Gynecomastia, Senescent Gynecomastia

These forms of gynecomastia represent physiological changes due to the respective hormonal situations. Breast imaging techniques play no role in the diagnostic work-up.

Gynecomastia

Pathological gynecomastia of the adult male develops under the influence of excess estrogen hormones or decreased levels of androgen hormones. In addition many drugs with an "estrogen-effect" have been found to cause gynecomastia. The following causes deserve special attention:

- Estrogen therapy, estrogen-secreting or human chorionic gonadotropin-secreting testicular or adrenal tumors, paraneoplastic syndrome, cirrhosis of the liver.
- Anorchism, castration, hypogonadism, Klinefelter syndrome, hyperthyroidism.
- Drugs including spironolactone, cimetidine, verapamil, marijuana.

MR mammography shows a hypointense retromamillary area in the T1-weighted precontrast sequence. After CM administration this area usually shows no or only slight contrast enhancement. If strong or suspicious contrast enhancement is found, biopsy must be performed to exclude malignancy.

Pseudogynecomastia

The enlarged breast in pseudogynecomastia contains only adipose tissue (overweight!) without evidence of parenchyma. Corresponding findings in MR mammography rule out true gynecomastia.

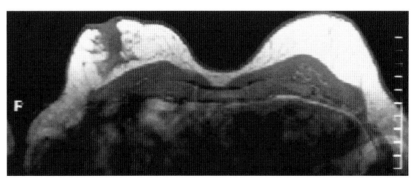

Fig. 10.**1 a, b   Unilateral gynecomastia.**
a   T1-weighted precontrast image shows parenchymal body in right retromamilllary region.

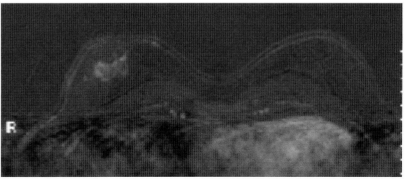

b   Subtraction image shows slight contrast enhancement.

Male Breast Cancer

In contrast to earlier opinion, there is no significant difference between the histology of male and female breast carcinoma. However, since tubular structures are not usually found in the male breast, there are only rare reports of male invasive lobular carcinoma. All other histological types of breast cancer (NOS, medullary, papillary, colloid, and Paget disease) have been reported in men, although the majority of tumors are infiltrating ductal carcinomas (Fig. 10.**2**).

Breast cancer in males is a rare disease representing less than 1 % of all breast cancers. The incidence of male breast cancer increases with age and shows a peak between the 50th and 70th years of life (0.1/100 000 for 35-year-olds; 11/100 000 for 85-year-olds).

Risk factors implicated in the increased incidence of male breast cancer include undescended testicles, orchitis, infertility, hypercholesteremia, exogenous estrogen administration, and radiation exposure (latent period 12–35 years). Approximately 30 % of men with breast cancer have a family history of the disease in female or male family members.

Primary diagnostic procedures performed when male breast cancer is suspected are mammography and percutaneous biopsy. Gynecomastia, which itself is not a risk factor for the development of breast cancer, must be considered as a differential diagnosis.

Findings on MR mammography are like those of female breast cancer and show the same characteristics of malignancy.

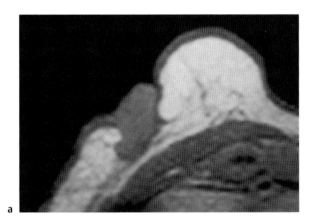

a

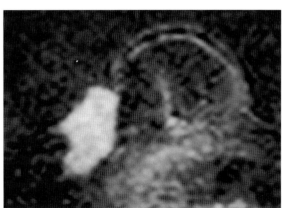

b

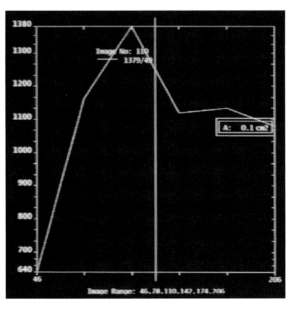

c

Fig. 10.**2 a–c Male breast cancer.**
a T1-weighted precontrast image shows a centrally located tumor with ulceration in the ventral portions.
b Subtraction image shows hypervascularized smooth-bordered, lobulated lesion.
c Signal intensity curve analysis shows strong initial contrast enhancement (>100 %) with postinitial „wash-out".
Histology: Invasive ductal carcinoma.

11 Indications for MR Mammography

MR Mammography in Patients with Ambiguous Findings

The combination of clinical examination, mammography, and percutaneous biopsy is still the basis of breast cancer diagnostics. Breast ultrasonography is a complementary diagnostic technique especially useful for the examination of breasts with mammographically dense parenchyma. Together, the findings derived from the clinical examination, imaging techniques, and cytological—i.e., histological—tests allow a comprehensive interpretation of breast lesions and changes (Table 11.**1** and Figs. 11.**1** and 11.**2**). Depending on the resulting evaluation, findings can then be assigned to one of five assessment categories: **Category 1 (no findings)** includes normal examination results without identification of notable findings. **Category 2 (definitely benign finding(s))** includes examination results with identifiable lesions, i.e., changes that are typically benign (e.g., lipoma, oil cyst, hamartoma, calcified fibroadenoma). **Category 3 (probably benign finding(s))** includes examination results with identifiable lesions, i.e., changes having a high probability of being benign (e.g., noncalcified fibroadenoma, focal mammographic densities due to overlap of parenchymal structures). **Category 4 (possibly malignant finding(s))** includes examination results with a suspicious abnormality that does not have typical characteristics of malignancy but requires further investigation. **Category 5 (finding(s) highly suggestive of malignancy)** includes examination results with identifiable lesions, i.e., changes having a very high probability of being malignant.

The comprehensive interpretation of breast findings must take the potential and limitations of each diagnostic examination into consideration. It does not require that all diagnostic techniques be performed in all cases, nor that breast lesions or changes be identifiable with all methods (e.g., clustered pleomorphic microcalcifications seen on mammography need not correlate with a palpable or ultrasonographic lesion to be highly suggestive of malignancy).

Dynamic MR mammography can occasionally be indicated in the diagnostic work-up of findings in assessment **category 3** if the conventional imaging techniques have been performed but have not allowed malignancy to be excluded with a high enough probability.

For findings in assessment **category 4**, MR mammography is performed as a complementary diagnostic examination. When all characteristics of malignancy are missing in the MRI examination, open biopsy may sometimes be averted (see Chapter 12). If MR mammo-

graphy cannot circumvent open biopsy, results are used as preoperative local staging.

MR mammography can play a significant role in the preoperative staging of patients with lesions highly suggestive of malignancy (**category 5**). Its value lies in the additional information it may provide pertaining to tumor size and extent, multicentricity, and bilaterality.

Numerous reports can be found in current literature pertaining to the use of MR mammography to further evaluate ambiguous findings in x-ray mammography and/or ultrasonography. These are often referred to as so-called "problem cases". Buchberger and co-workers perform MR mammography as a complementary technique for ambiguous localized lesions and diffuse abnormalities, and have been able to show that MR mammography provides additional diagnostic information in some cases. They do not, however, recommend refraining from biopsy (Buchberger et al. 1997). Gilles and colleagues. emphasize the high sensitivity (95%) of MR mammography for clinically occult lesions, but the specificity in this study only reached 53% (Gilles et al. 1994). Heywang-Köbrunner and co-workers. demonstrated that the performance of MR mammography in a patient collective of 525 "problem cases" increased sensitivity from 60% to 98% and specificity from 45% to 65%. It must be noted, however, that the collective in this study included studies performed in search of an unknown primary tumor, and postoperatively, which are both already accepted indications for the performance of MR mammography (Heywang-Köbrunner et al. 1990). Rieber and colleagues have shown in a retrospective analysis that a normal MR mammogram performed for further evaluation of an ambiguous breast lesion correctly rules out malignancy in over 96% of cases. Both invasive (0.8%) and intraductal (2.9%) lesions were missed, however (Rieber et al. 1997).

In summary, the studies published in the current literature are burdened by the fact that often not all indicated conventional diagnostic procedures were performed. Descriptions of ultrasonographic findings were occasionally missing and, in most cases, no mention was made of a percutaneous biopsy. To evaluate the importance of dynamic MR mammography, especially with consideration of cost-effectiveness for the respective indications, prospective studies defining specific "problem cases" must be performed.

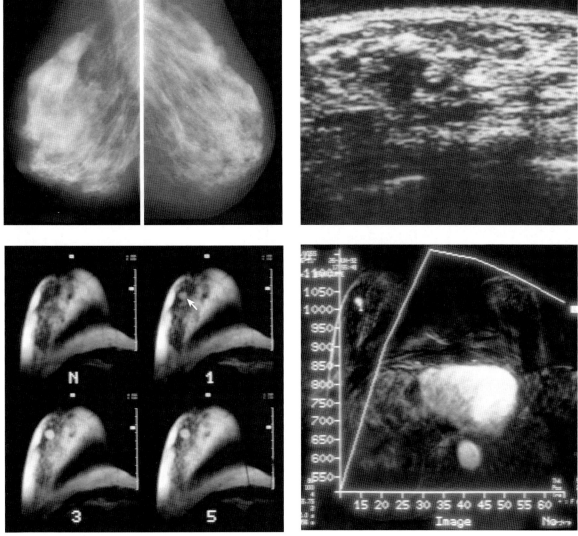

Fig. 11.**1a–d   MR mammography performed for further evaluation of an ambiguous finding.** 81-year-old patient. No hormone replacement therapy. Ambiguous palpable lump laterally of the right nipple.

a Mammography shows heterogeneously dense breast tissue (ACR type 3) without identifiable lesion.
b Ultrasonography reveals an ill-defined, hypoechoic lesion in the upper outer quadrant of the right breast.
c Dynamic MR mammography with normal findings in precontrast examination. Postcontrast examination shows hy-

pervascularized, smooth-bordered, round lesion with ring-enhancement in the right upper outer quadrant (arrow).
d Signal analysis shows strong initial contrast enhancement with postinitial wash-out phenomenon.
Ultrasound (US)-guided large-core biopsy: no evidence of malignancy.
Interpretation: Suspicious abnormality in the right breast.
Consequence: Open biopsy after preoperative US-guided localization of lesion in the right upper outer quadrant.
Histology: Invasive ductal carcinoma pT1c (12 mm) GII N0.

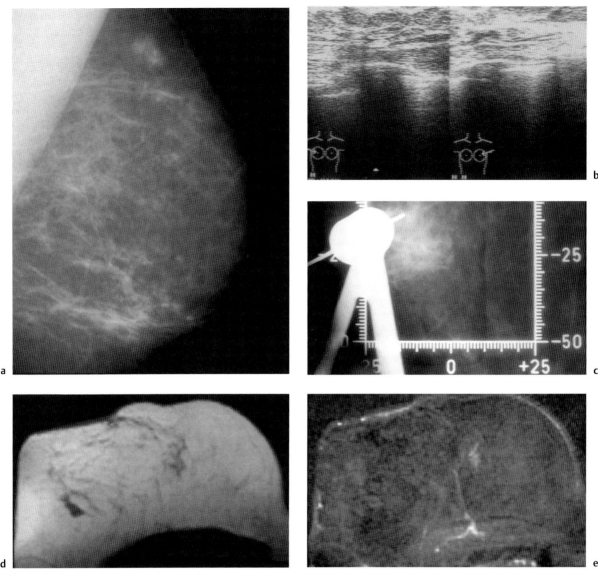

Fig. 11.**2 a–e MR mammography performed for further evaluation of an ambiguous finding.** 56-year-old patient. Screening mammogram. No high risk factors. Normal findings upon clinical examination.

a Mammography shows fibroglandular breast tissue (ACR type 2) with an ill-defined lesion in the upper outer quadrant of right breast.

b No identifiable correlating lesion on ultrasonography.

c Histology after stereotactic large-core biopsy: proliferative fibrocystic changes of the breast without atypia.

d T1-weighted precontrast image shows corresponding finding.

e Subtraction image shows no contrast enhancement in ambiguous region (second measurement after contrast administration).

Interpretation: Probably benign finding in the right breast.

Consequence: Follow-up mammography in six months.

Follow-up showed unchanging mammographic findings over four years.

Table 11.**1**   Indication for MR Mammography Depending upon Comprehensive Interpretation after Conventional Diagnostics

Comprehensive Interpretation	Category	Consequence
Negative	1	No MRI
Benign finding	2	No MRI
Probably benign finding	3	! MRI
Suspicious abnormality	4	! MRI
Highly suggestive of malignancy	5	MRI staging

Indication for MR mammography: Ambiguous breast findings

MR mammography can provide additional, relevant diagnostic information in patients with an ambiguous breast finding after the performance of conventional imaging techniques or when for some reason these cannot be performed. This is especially true for ambiguous lesions between 5 and 10 mm in diameter.

Cave
MR mammography should not be performed to further evaluate suspicious microcalcifications since these may indicate the presence of intraductal breast cancer, which cannot be reliably confirmed or excluded by MRI (see Chapter 9, DCIS).

Preoperative Staging

The preoperative performance of MR mammography is one of the most important indications for its use. Of all breast imaging techniques, it is the one with the greatest sensitivity for the detection of invasive mammary tumors. It is for this reason that MR mammography is especially suitable to give additional preoperative information about the tumor extent, possible multifocality or multicentricity, as well as the presence of contralateral breast cancer. Studies published to date convincingly document the effectiveness of preoperative MR staging in the planning of the appropriate stage-dependent treatment strategy.

Tumor Size

Studies comparing the preoperative estimation of tumor size by breast imaging techniques (mammography, ultrasonography, MR mammography) with histological tumor measurements prove that MR mammography is superior to the other modalities. Boetes et al. (1995) found no significant difference in the size estimated by MR mammography and that measured in the histological specimen. In contrast, mammography (14% deviation) and ultrasonography (18% deviation) significantly underestimated tumor size. These results are corroborated by those of Mumtaz et al. (1997) ($r^2 = 0.93$ for MR mammography, $r^2 = 0.59$ for x-ray mammography) and Rodenko et al. (1996) (85% for MR mammography vs. 32% for x-ray mammography).

Extensive Intraductal Component (EIC)

MR mammography is also superior to conventional x-ray mammography in the detection of an intraductal tumor component (Figs. 11.**3** and 11.**5**). In this regard, Mumtaz and colleagues have shown a sensitivity of 81% and a specificity of 93% for MR mammography, whereas the respective values for x-ray mammography (62% and 74%) are significantly lower (Mumtaz et al. 1997). In agreement, Soderstrom and colleagues have reported the correct estimation of tumor extent in preoperative MR mammography in 95% of cases (vs. x-ray mammography in 74% of cases) (Soderstrom et al 1996).

The principal characteristic in MR mammography indicating the presence of an EIC is a contrast-enhancing area with dendritic configuration adjacent to the primary tumor. The additional presence of small round or ovoid enhancing foci is often a sign indicating microinvasive tumor. Due to the dendritic configuration of the extensive intraductal component in MR mammography, selected ROIs for the signal analysis are very small and the signal–time curves obtained often lack the typical characteristics indicating malignancy. In the presence of the morphological changes described above, therefore, an unsuspicious signal–time curve cannot rule out an EIC.

Multifocality

Many definitions of *multifocality* can be found in the medical literature. Most groups base their accounts on the interpretation of Lagios and colleagues, defining multifocality as the presence of two or more lesions within one quadrant of the breast (Lagios et al. 1981).

> **Multifocality**
> **Two or more carcinomas within one breast quadrant.**

The reported incidence of multifocal breast cancer (Figs. 11.**4** and 11.**7**) varies between 25% and 50%. The mammographic detection rate of multifocality is ~15%.

In our own patient collective, ~8% of breast carcinomas were shown to be multifocal. Over 70% of these were recognized preoperatively as such solely in MR mammography (Fischer et al. 1999). These results accord with those of other groups (Rieber et al. 1997; Harms et al. 1993).

Multicentricity

The definition of *multicentricity* also varies. It is recommended that a strict definition be applied that describes the assignment of multiple lesions to breast quadrants and requires that secondary lesions have a certain minimum distance from the primary lesion.

> **Multicentricity**
> **One or more carcinomas present in a breast quadrant other than the one that harbored the primary lesion, and having a minimum distance of 2 cm from this lesion.**

There is great discrepancy in the reported incidence of multicentric breast cancer (Fig. 11.**6**) due to the use of different definitions. Histopathological studies have reported values between 40% and 60%. It must be mentioned, however, that some of the histologically proven intraductal lesions leading to the diagnosis of multicentricity will not progress to symptomatic invasive cancers and are therefore clinically insignificant. Realistic estimations of the incidence of multicentricity appear to be between 15% and 30%.

Several studies have demonstrated MR mammography to be the most sensitive method for detecting the presence of breast cancer multicentricity. Our own pre-

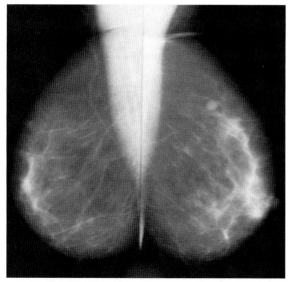
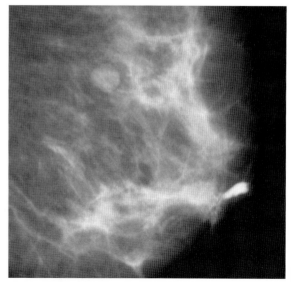

a

b

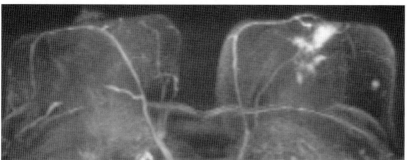

c

Fig. 11.**3 a–c Mammary carcinoma with EIC.** 54-year-old patient. Bloody nipple discharge from left breast. No abnormal palpable findings.

a Mammography shows asymmetric breast tissue density (ACR type 1 on right, ACR type 2 on left). Ill-defined hyperdensity in left retromamillary region containing suspicious microcalcifications.

b Galactography shows dilated duct ending bluntly at microcalcification cluster.

Exfoliative cytology: Carcinoma cells.

Comprehensive interpretation: Mammary carcinoma of the left breast.

c Confirmation of tumor in MR mammography (MIP technique). Additional documentation of dendritic contrast enhancement extending toward the central portion of the breast. Side finding: Fibroadenoma in lateral portion of left breast.

Histology: Ductal carcinoma (pT1c) with EIC.

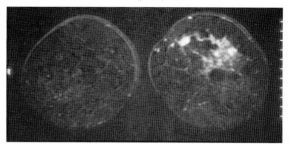

b

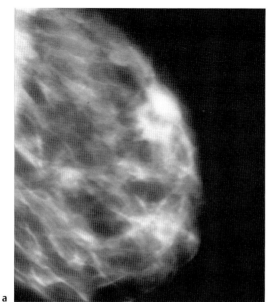

a

Fig. 11.**4 a, b Multifocal mammary carcinoma.** 48-year-old patient. Palpable tumor in upper inner quadrant of left breast.

a Mammography shows heterogenously dense breast tissue (ACR type 3) with an ill-defined lesion.

Identification of correlating lesion in ultrasonography (no figure).

Comprehensive interpretation: Lesion highly suggestive of malignancy.

b MR mammography subtraction image confirms corresponding lesion with characteristics typical of malignancy. Additional documentation of tumor extension far laterally (coronal angulation).

Histology: Multifocal, partly ductal invasive, partly mucinous breast carcinoma pT1c GII N0 (0/10).

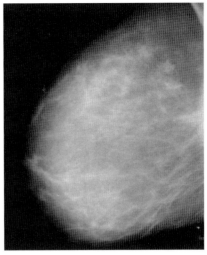
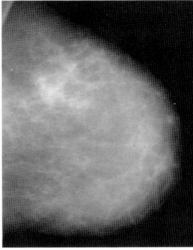

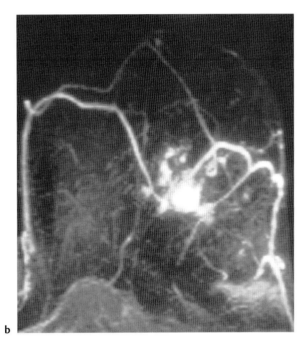

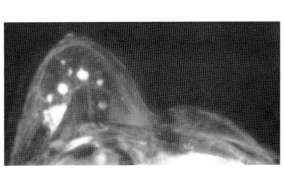

Fig. 11.**5 a,b** **Mammary carcinoma with EIC.** 50-year-old patient. Palpable tumor in central portion of left breast.
a Mammography shows fibroglandular breast tissue (ACR type 2) with an ill-defined lesion in the central-lateral area of the left breast.
Comprehensive interpretation: Left lesion highly suggestive of malignancy.
b MR mammography shows a hypervascularized lesion in the central portion of the left breast with partly dendritic, partly round contrast enhancing areas adjacent to tumor as sign of intraductal—i.e., microinvasive—tumor component (MIP technique).
Histology: Invasive ductal breast cancer (pT1c [11 mm] GIII) with extensive DCIS manifestation and microinvasive areas in the periphery (solid subtype, GIII).

Fig. 11.**6 a, b** **Multicentric mammary carcinoma.** 41-year-old patient. Postmastectomy status left. Palpable abnormality in lower portion of right breast.
a Mammography shows heterogenously dense breast tissue (ACR type 3) with an ill-defined lesion (arrow).
Comprehensive interpretation: Lesion highly suggestive of malignancy.
b MR mammography confirms an oval lesion in the lower outer quadrant and additionally depicts further hypervascularized lesions in all quadrants as evidence of multicentric tumor growth.
Histology: Multicentric ductal invasive breast carcinoma (pT2 GII).   ▽

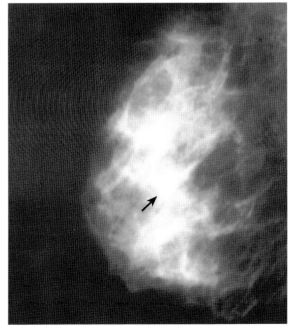

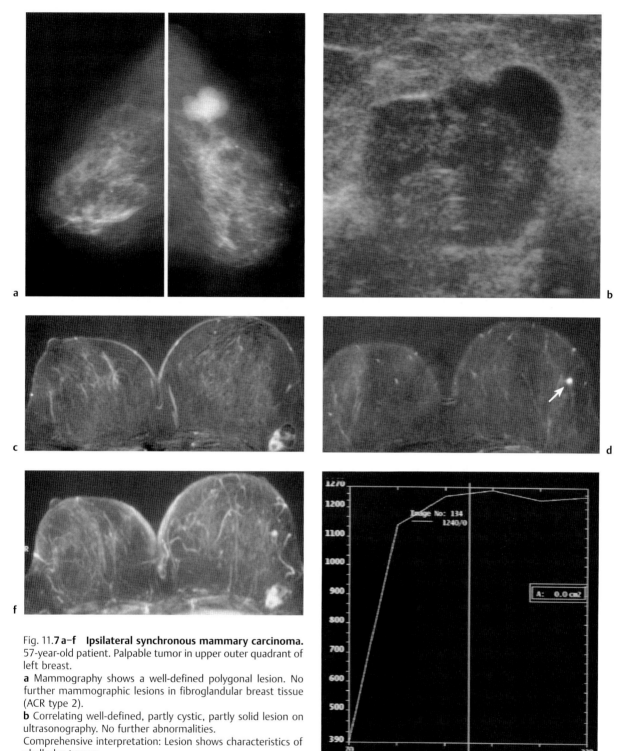

Fig. 11.**7 a–f** **Ipsilateral synchronous mammary carcinoma.**
57-year-old patient. Palpable tumor in upper outer quadrant of
left breast.
a Mammography shows a well-defined polygonal lesion. No
further mammographic lesions in fibroglandular breast tissue
(ACR type 2).
b Correlating well-defined, partly cystic, partly solid lesion on
ultrasonography. No further abnormalities.
Comprehensive interpretation: Lesion shows characteristics of
phyllodes tumor.
c Preoperative MR mammography: single slice subtraction
image shows a partially hypervascularized, well-defined lesion
in the upper outer quadrant of the left breast.
d Documentation of small additional hypervascularized lesion
of 5 mm diameter (arrow) in the lower outer quadrant of the
left breast.
e Signal analysis of additionally detected lesion (**d**) shows very
strong initial contrast enhancement with postinitial plateau.
f Depiction of both lesions in MIP technique.

Course of action: Surgical excision of palpable tumor and second smaller lesion (after preoperative MR localization).

Histology: Malignant phyllodes tumor of 3 cm diameter in the
upper outer quadrant of the left breast. Invasive ductal carcinoma (pT1a [5 mm] GII) in the lower outer quadrant of the left
breast.

operative MRI studies on a large collective of patients (n = 463) show that multicentric tumors are found in about 12% of breast cancer patients. In half of these cases, multicentricity was detected solely in MR mammography (Fischer et al. 1999). These results are confirmed by studies on smaller patient collectives by other groups. Rieber et al. (1997) found bifocal carcinomas solely by MR mammography in 11% of cases; Oellinger et al. (1993) in 28% of cases; and Harms et al. (1993) in 37% of cases.

Synchronous Bilateral Breast Cancer

Reports document that the synchronous presentation of bilateral breast cancer (Fig. 11.**8**) occurs in ~5% of all breast cancer patients. The incidence of bilateral invasive lobular carcinoma is reported to be significantly higher (up to 30%).

In our own preoperative MRI studies, a synchronous contralateral carcinoma was found in 5% of breast cancer patients (Fischer et al. 1994). Rieber et al. (1997) preoperatively examined 34 patients with a histologically verified mammary carcinoma and obtained identical results. In addition, it was shown that 75% of synchronous contralateral carcinomas can only be detected by MR mammography (Fischer et al. 1999).

N Staging

MR mammography does not allow a reliable statement pertaining to metastatic axillary lymph node involvement (Rodenko et al 1996). On the one hand, unspecific enhancement, e.g., inflammatory lymph node reaction, may lead to false-positive findings. On the other, micrometastases (pN1a) do not necessarily show a pathological contrast enhancement (false-negative).

MR Mammographic Consequences for Therapeutic Strategy

The primary treatment of breast cancer is based on its surgical excision. It must be decided preoperatively whether breast-conserving therapy is an option. Criteria making local excision (tumorectomy, lumpectomy) less advisable or impossible are large tumor size (usually over 2–3 cm, case reports up to 5 cm), unfavorable size of the tumor relative to the breast, and the presence of multicentric tumors. Naturally, the wishes of the informed patient must also be considered. Adjuvant therapies are radiation therapy and/or various combination chemotherapies.

The additional diagnostic information provided by preoperative MR mammography altered the surgical procedures performed in 14% of patients in our own collective. This applied in particular to the performance of a mastectomy instead of lumpectomy for multifocal and multicentric tumors, and to the performance of a contralateral lumpectomy for otherwise occult breast cancer (Fischer et al. 1994, 1999). Orel and colleagues

also reported a change in the therapeutic strategy for 11% of breast cancer patients due to the additional information provided by the preoperative MR mammography (Orel et al. 1995).

In contrast, in 3–5% of patients the preoperative MR mammography results in false-positive findings, leading to an "unnecessary" extension of the surgical procedure (Fischer et al. 1994; Rieber et al. 1997).

When the indication is appropriate for the performance of MR mammography, this examination is relatively cost-effective, especially considering the independent necessity for surgery and connected hospital stay. In this context, the rate of false-positive findings and the consequent alteration of surgical procedures appears acceptable. In most cases there is neither a separate surgical risk nor an increased hospital stay for the patient.

Indication for MR mammography: Preoperative staging

MR mammography is indicated for women with a clinical and/or mammographic and/or sonographic lesion suspicious for or typical of malignancy (categories 4 and 5), which necessitates an open biopsy for histological verification. As can be expected, additional diagnostic information is obtained primarily for women with heterogeneously and extremely dense parenchyma (ACR types 3 and 4). On the other hand, if the breast is composed entirely or almost entirely of fat (ACR type 1), a preoperative MRI staging of the breast can often be forgone. It is important that when otherwise occult lesions are detected on MR mammography, the performance of a preoperative MR-guided localization should be possible.

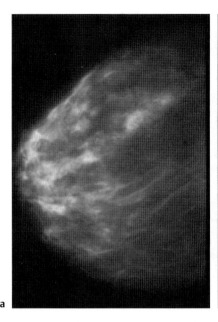
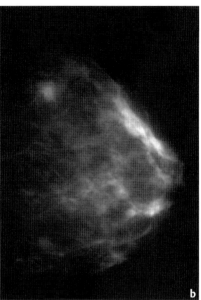
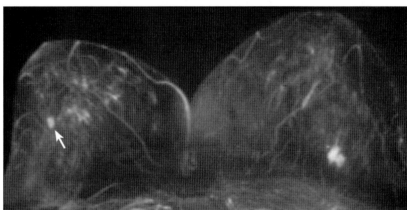

Fig. 11.**8 a–e   Synchronous bilateral breast cancer.** 61-year-old patient. Palpable tumor in upper outer quadrant of left breast.

a, b   Mammography shows heterogenously dense breast tissue (ACR type 3) with a suspicious lesion in the left breast corresponding to palpable finding. Contralateral mammography of the right breast shows heterogenously dense breast tissue (ACR type 3) without a distinct lesion.
Comprehensive interpretation: Left lesion suspicious of malignancy.

c   MR mammography subtraction image confirms twin lesion in the left breast showing characteristics typical of malignancy. Additional documentation of an 8 mm partially ill-defined hypervascularized lesion in the right breast (arrow).

d   Signal–time curve of the right lesion.

e   Signal–time curve of the left lesion.

Course of action: Surgical excision of palpable left tumor and right lesion after preoperative MR localization.

Histology: Multifocal, ductal invasive breast carcinoma (pT2 GII) of the left breast, and invasive ductal carcinoma (pT1b [7 mm] GII) of the right breast.

Neoadjuvant Chemotherapy

The expression *neoadjuvant chemotherapy* is used to denote primary cytostatic therapy before surgical intervention. In the past, this therapeutic strategy was predominantly applied to inflammatory breast cancer because this tumor form cannot usually be adequately surgically excised. In recent years, neoadjuvant chemotherapy has also been used increasingly in the therapy of locally advanced breast cancer, especially in younger women.

In the course of chemotherapy, clinical, ultrasonographic, and mammographic examinations are of limited use in providing information on the tumor response. Because MR mammography provides information pertaining to tumor size and vascularization, it has proven to be a very useful sectional imaging technique in therapy response monitoring during the course of neoadjuvant chemotherapy (Fig. 11.**9**). Its greatest value lies in the differentiation between "responders" and "nonresponders".

! **MRI criteria for sensitiveness of tumor to chemotherapy (so-called responders)**
- Reduction of tumor size by more than 25 %
- Flattening of initial ascent in signal–time curve
- Decrease of maximum contrast enhancement

According to Rieber et al. (1997), the initial contrast enhancement of responder tumors is higher than that of nonresponder tumors at the time of diagnosis. Gilles and colleagues reported 18 patients whose tumors showed a good correlation between contrast enhancement within the tumor and histopathological findings after neoadjuvant therapy. These authors remark, however, on the possibility of false-negative findings due to small residual intraductal tumor and invasive tumors few millimeters in size (Gilles et al. 1994). These observations have been confirmed by Rieber et al. (1997) and Kurtz et al. (1996). Knopp and colleagues have demonstrated typical signal–time curves for patients with tumors that did not respond, partially responded, and responded well to neoadjuvant chemotherapy using several example cases (Knopp et al. 1994; Junkermann and von Fournier 1997).

**Indication for MR mammography:
Therapy response monitoring of neoadjuvant chemotherapy**

When neoadjuvant chemotherapy is planned, MR mammography should be performed before therapy to ascertain and document the pretherapeutic MRI status. The first evaluation examination as part of therapy response monitoring is performed after the second cycle of chemotherapy. The results of this examination are the basis for the decision whether chemotherapy should be continued (responder) or not (nonresponder). The next evaluation examination is performed after the fourth cycle of chemotherapy, if applicable.

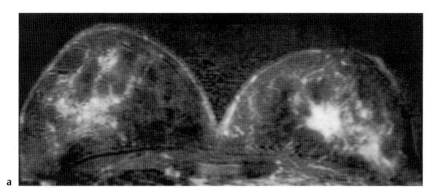

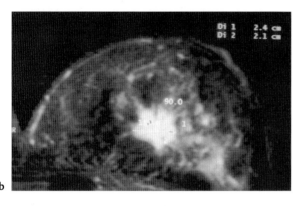

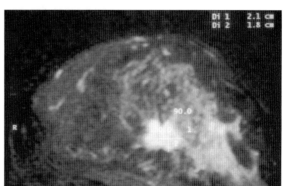

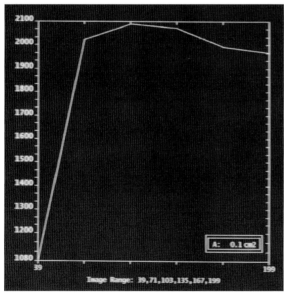

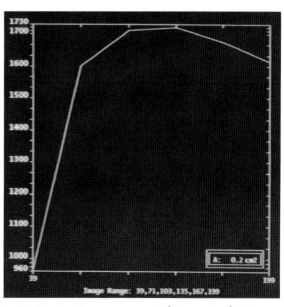

Fig. 11.**9 a–e** **Therapy response monitoring of neoadjuvant chemotherapy for breast cancer.** 39-year-old patient. Histologically verified invasive ductal mammary carcinoma GII.

a MIP image before beginning chemotherapy. Documentation of tumor within diffusely enhancing parenchyma of the left breast.

b Semiquantitative measurement of tumor size before chemotherapy (5 cm²).

c Semiquantitative measurement of tumor size after two cycles of chemotherapy (3.8 cm²).

d Signal–time curve before beginning chemotherapy

e Signal–time curve after two cycles of chemotherapy. Slight flattening of initial ascent from 48 % to 43 %.

Carcinoma of Unknown Primary (CUP Syndrome)

CUP syndrome denotes the presence of metastases without knowledge of the primary tumor site from which these originate. A typical constellation in breast diagnostics is the detection of an axillary lymph node metastasis without prior identification of the related primary tumor (e.g., in the breast).

❗ Common sites of metastatic spread from breast cancer
- Lymphogenous spread: locoregional (especially axillary, clavicular, and parasternal lymph node)
- Hematogenous spread: to bone, lung, liver, and brain

Mammography is the diagnostic imaging method of choice in such a setting. Ultrasonography of the breast is a useful complementary method. Dynamic MR mammography is indicated when both these diagnostic techniques have failed to identify an intramammary primary tumor (Fig. 11.**10**).

Reports in the literature reveal an unexpectedly high rate of success in identifying the primary tumor for CUP syndrome with dynamic MR mammography when performed for specific indications. In our own study, dynamic MR mammography was performed in 14 patients with metastases of unknown primary tumors (lymph node metastases: 6 axillary, 1 supraclavicular, 1 inguinal; 1 bone metastasis; 3 liver metastases; 1 lung metastasis), and normal findings of the breast in clinical, mammographic, and ultrasonographic examinations. The primary mammary carcinoma was detected in six cases. False-positive findings were found in three cases (fibroadenoma, sclerosing adenosis). In the remaining five patients with normal MR mammographic findings, follow-up confirmed that no breast cancer was present (Schorn et al. 1997). Morris et al. (1997) studied 12 patients with axillary lymph node metastases and found the primary mammary carcinoma in nine cases solely in MR mammography. Similar results are reported by the groups of Porter (Porter et al. 1995) of and Van Die (Van Die et al. 1996).

Indication for MR mammography: CUP syndrome

MR mammography is indicated for women with normal findings in clinical, mammographic, and ultrasonographic examinations of the breast in the following situations:
- Presence of lymph node metastases histologically consistent with a mammary carcinoma (especially axillary lymph node).
- Presence of bone, lung, liver, or brain metastases histologically consistent with a mammary carcinoma.
- Presence of a metastasis constellation that makes a primary mammary carcinoma seem probable.

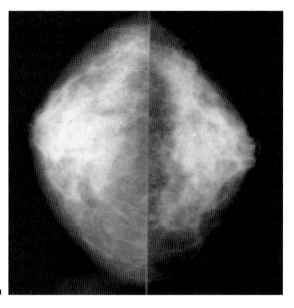
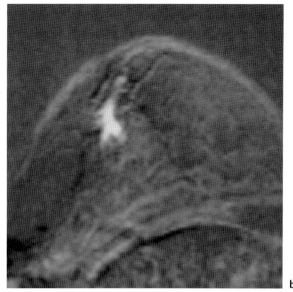

a

b

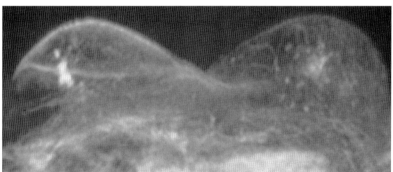
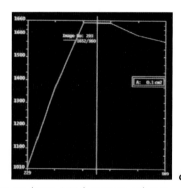

c

d

Fig. 11.**10 a–d** **CUP syndrome.** 58-year-old patient with bone metastases from unknown primary tumor.

a Mammography shows extremely dense breast tissue (ACR type 4) without definable lesion.

b MR mammography shows dendritic contrast enhancement in the right retromamillary region (single slice subtraction image).

c Documentation of findings in MIP technique.

d Signal analysis shows moderate initial contrast enhancement with postinitial plateau.

Course of action: Surgical excision of lesion after preoperative MR localization.

Histology: Invasive ductal breast carcinoma (pT1c [16 mm] pN0 M1 GII).

Differentiation between Scar and Carcinoma

Differentiation between a postoperative scar (Fig. 11.**12**) and a malignant tumor (Fig. 11.**11**) is an important application of MR mammography since the administration of contrast material yields a visual representation of the vascular conditions in the breast. Once the healing of a wound is completed, the differentiation between non-vascularized scar tissue and strongly vascularized tumor is, therefore, very reliable.

All groups of workers unanimously report an extremely high sensitivity of MR mammography for the verification of scar tissue. Our experience is that localized enhancing areas within or in the vicinity of a scar must arouse the suspicion of malignancy even when signal analysis yields an unspecific signal–time curve. Apparently, tumor angiogenesis does not always reach advanced development in carcinomas within fibrotic scar tissue. The main differential diagnosis of such localized enhancing areas is a localized inflammatory process within the scar tissue. The reactive hyperemia it causes can imitate the findings of a malignant tumor in MRI. The absence of contrast enhancement rules out an invasive tumor process with high reliability.

> **! Cave:**
> The required interval between open biopsy and MR mammography is six months

> **Indication for MR mammography: Differentiation between scar and carcinoma**
>
> MR mammography is indicated when x-ray mammography and ultrasonography cannot reliably differentiate between a postoperative scar and carcinoma.

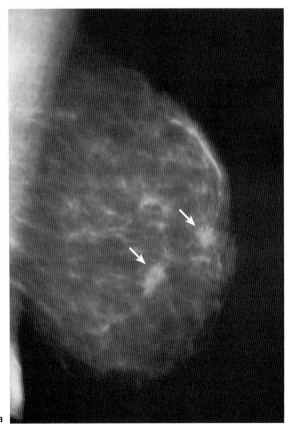

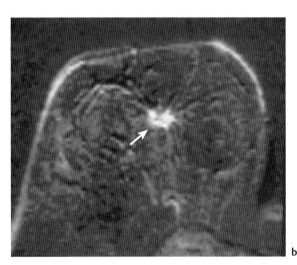

Fig. 11.**11 a, b** **Carcinoma in postoperative scar.** 63-year-old patient. Postoperative scar in right breast after ductectomy two years earlier.
a Mammography shows two spiculated lesions in the retro-mamillary (i.e., central) region (arrows).
   Comprehensive interpretation: Lesions suspicious of malignancy (differential diagnosis: scar tissue).
b MR mammography (subtraction image) shows prominent contrast enhancement in central spiculated lesion (arrow). No contrast enhancement in the second retromamillary lesion.
Histology: central invasive ductal breast carcinoma (pT1b [6 mm] N0 GIII), retromamillary scar.

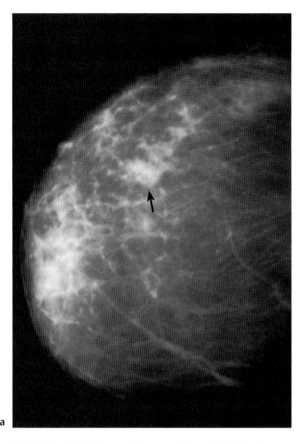

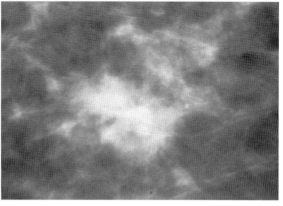

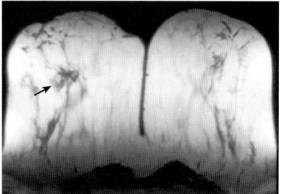

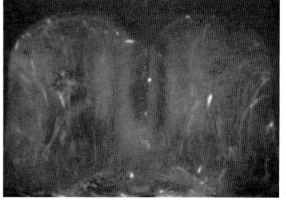

Fig. 11.**12 a–d   Postoperative scar.** 46-year-old patient.

a First postoperative mammography examination after open biopsy of the right breast three years earlier. Within fibro-glandular breast tissue (ACR type 2) identification of ill-defined irregularly bordered hyperdensity without microcalcifications (arrow).

b Partial magnification from contact image. No correlating lesion on ultrasonography (no figure)
Comprehensive interpretation: Scar or carcinoma.

c Identification of correlating lesion in T1-weighted precontrast image (arrow).

d Subtraction image shows no contrast enhancement. Final diagnosis: postoperative scar.

Follow-up mammography over four years showed no changes.

Follow-up after Lumpectomy

The diagnostic value of x-ray mammography and ultrasonography is known to be limited after breast-conserving surgery and adjuvant radiotherapy for breast cancer. As already discussed, MR mammography represents the most reliable imaging method for the early detection of intramammary recurrences of breast cancer (Figs. 11.**13**–11.**15**).

> **⚠ Note:**
> Interval between end of radiotherapy after lumpectomy and MR mammography should be 12 months
>
> **Cave:**
> Contrast enhancement after radiotherapy varies greatly between individuals.

There is agreement in the experience of various groups of the value of MR mammography in the follow-up examinations after lumpectomy: tumor recurrences show a prominent enhancement within the first minutes after contrast administration, whereas scar tissue shows no contrast enhancement. Various groups report a sensitivity of MR mammography for the detection of tumor recurrences of up to 100% (Heywang-Köbrunner et al. 1990; Krämer et al. 1998). The reported incidence of MR mammographically detected recurrences ranges from 10% to 25%. On the average these are discovered 2–3 years after lumpectomy and have range in size from 5 to 15 mm. In addition, Rieber and colleagues have shown that mammographically and/or ultrasonographically suspicious lesions after lumpectomy are proven to be true negative findings on MR mammography in a high percentage of cases. Due to the MR mammographic findings, further diagnostic procedures can be avoided for these patients (Rieber et al. 1997). Furthermore, in cases where tumor recurrence has been verified, MR mammography allows an evaluation of the breast near the chest wall and an assessment of possible tumor infiltration of the pectoral muscle.

> **Indication for MR mammography:**
> **Differentiation between tumor recurrence and posttherapeutic effects**
>
> MR mammography is indicated when x-ray mammography and ultrasonography cannot reliably rule out a tumor recurrence after lumpectomy with or without adjuvant radiotherapy. There are no defined recommendations for MRI follow-up intervals. Especially for patients with dense parenchyma limiting the sensitivity of x-ray mammography (ACR types 3 and 4), MR mammography seems advisable in the second or third year after lumpectomy, and at intervals of, say, two years thereafter.

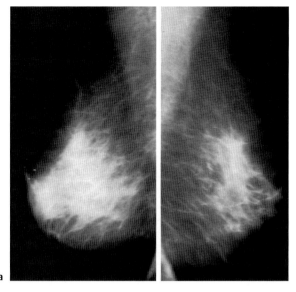

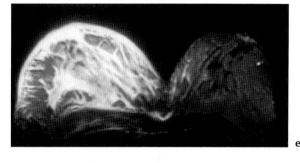

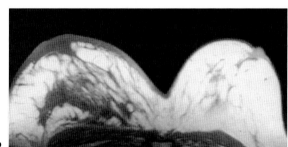

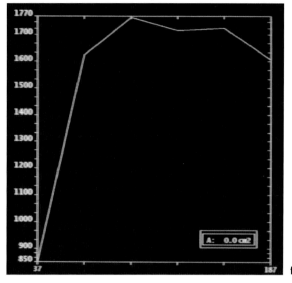

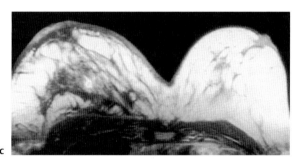

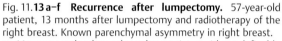

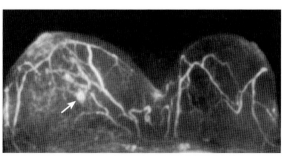

Fig. 11.**13 a–f Recurrence after lumpectomy.** 57-year-old patient, 13 months after lumpectomy and radiotherapy of the right breast. Known parenchymal asymmetry in right breast.

a Mammography shows dense breast tissue without definable lesion. Ultrasonography also revealed no definable lesion (no figure).

b T1-weighted precontrast image shows skin thickening of the right breast.

c Postcontrast image shows an ill-defined, ring shaped enhancing lesion in the central portion of the right breast. Moderate contrast enhancement in the skin of the right breast.

d Documentation of suspicious lesion in MIP technique (arrow).

e T2-weighted image shows prominent edematous changes throughout the right breast as a consequence of radiotherapy. No demarcation of a suspicious lesion.

f Signal analysis shows strong initial contrast enhancement with postinitial plateau.

Course of action: Surgical excision of lesion after preoperative MR localization.

Histology: Invasive ductal breast carcinoma (pT1b GII).

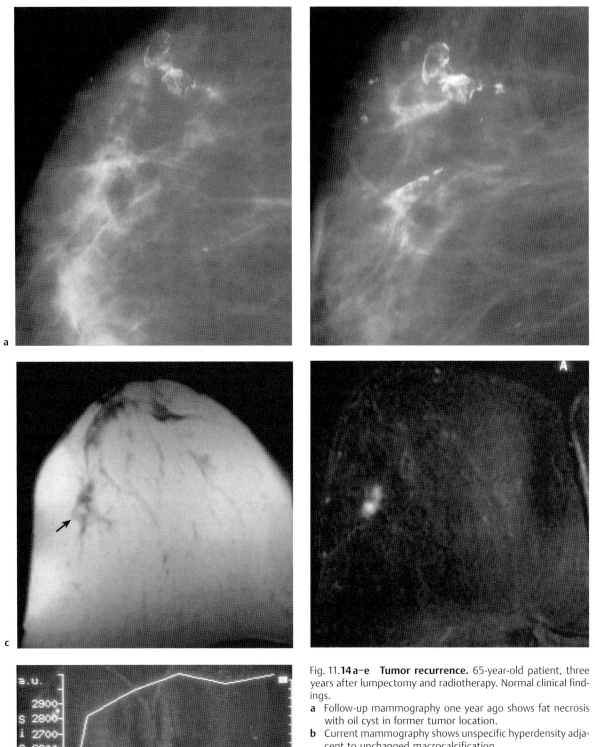

Fig. 11.**14 a–e** **Tumor recurrence.** 65-year-old patient, three years after lumpectomy and radiotherapy. Normal clinical findings.

a Follow-up mammography one year ago shows fat necrosis with oil cyst in former tumor location.

b Current mammography shows unspecific hyperdensity adjacent to unchanged macrocalcification.

c T1-weighted precontrast image shows signal-intense lesion correlating with oil cyst (arrow).

d Subtraction image shows dumbbell-shaped hypervascularized area neighboring oil cyst.

e Signal analysis shows slight initial contrast enhancement with postinitial plateau.

Histology: Invasive ductal breast cancer recurrence ([12 mm] GII) next to oil cyst.

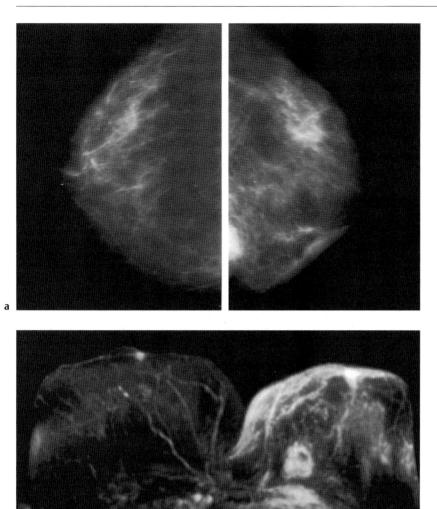

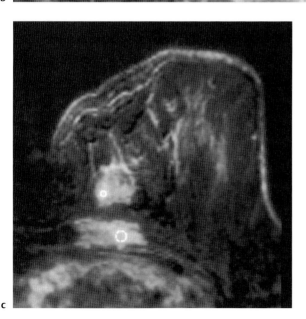

Fig. 11.15 a–c   Infiltration of thoracic wall by breast cancer recurrence after lumpectomy. 60-year-old patient, two years after lumpectomy and radiotherapy of the left breast. Unchanged skin thickening, no palpable abnormality.

a Mammography in the cranio-caudal view partially depicts a lesion in the medial portion of the left breast close to the thoracic wall. Incomplete projection in other mammographic views. Skin thickening after radiotherapy.

Comprehensive interpretation: Breast cancer recurrence.

b MR mammography confirms a hypervascularized lesion in medial portion of the left breast. In addition, the MIP image shows local tumor infiltration of the pectoral muscle. Note summation effect due to enhancement of skin in several slices.

c Documentation of findings in single slice subtraction image.
Histology (large-core biopsy): Recurrence of invasive ductal breast carcinoma.

Follow-up after Breast Reconstruction with Implant

The diagnostic value of conventional imaging techniques is very limited for patients with breast implants. This is true both for the evaluation with regard to prostheses complications and for the detection of periprosthetic and retroprosthetic carcinomas. Specific sequence protocols are employed for the MRI examination performed to answer the question of possible prosthesis complications (see Chapter 13). MR mammography to rule out malignancy is performed in the usual dynamic form using contrast material.

The retroprosthetic portions of the breast in particular, near the thoracic wall, cannot be adequately evaluated by mammography and ultrasonography. MR mammography in axial or sagittal slice orientation, on the other hand, can evaluate these areas well. However, the lateral portion of a prosthesis is occasionally overlapped by cardiac artifacts when performing the examination with the usual, medio-laterally directed, phase-encoding gradient (see Chapter 6). For this reason, it is recommended that an additional measurement be performed with a rotated phase-encoding gradient (90° rotation, ventro-dorsal direction) before the precontrast and immediately after finishing the dynamic examination (Fig. 11.**16**). If the subtraction of these two sequences reveals an enhancing area in the lateral periprosthetic or retroprosthetic potions of the breast, then an additional MRI examination with a phase-encoding gradient in the ventro-dorsal direction may be performed on one of the following days. This makes possible an adequate analysis of the signal–time curve.

Boné and colleagues found a breast cancer recurrence following mastectomy and breast reconstruction with implant in 17% of 83 patients. MR mammography was superior in this respect to clinical examination and x-ray mammography, detecting 12/14 recurrences (clinical 6/14, mammography 9/14). Since MRI missed two recurrences (false-negative findings, one of which was a DCIS), the combination of all three methods is recommended for the examination of patients with breast implants (Boné et al. 1995). Heinig and colleagues reported 13 recurrences in 169 patients following breast cancer treatment and reconstruction with implant. Twelve of these were detected on MR mammography, whereas the combined use of clinical examination, x-ray mammography, and ultrasonography detected only eight of these lesions. This study additionally showed that false-positive findings, usually caused by diffusely enhancing reactive inflammatory changes and focally enhancing granulomas, occurred most frequently in MRI examinations (Heinig et al. 1997). A careful analysis of the signal–time curve is therefore necessary to differentiate malignant from inflammatory changes, the latter rarely displaying a postinitial wash-out and only occasionally a plateau phase.

> **Indication for MR mammography:**
> **Follow-up after mastectomy and breast reconstruction with implant**
>
> MR mammography should be performed at regular intervals of 1–2 years as part of the diagnostic follow-up for women after mastectomy and breast reconstruction with implant. It is not usually indicated during the 12 months after insertion of an implant.

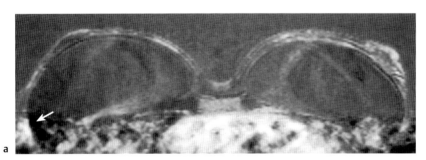

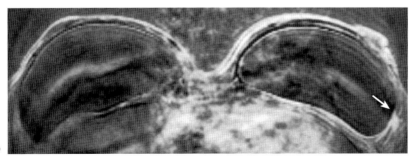

Fig. 11.**16 a, b   Recurrence following breast reconstruction with implant.** 40-year-old patient, two years after bilateral subcutaneous mastectomy (multifocal DCIS) and breast reconstruction with implant.
a MR mammography with medio-laterally directed phase-encoding gradient does not allow evaluation of lateral prosthesis portions. False enhancement lateral of right prosthesis due to cardiac artifacts (arrow).
b Examination in the late phase with a rotated phase-encoding gradient in the ventro-dorsal direction. Documentation of truly enhancing lesion lateral of the left prosthesis (arrow). As expected, stronger motion artifacts in the subtraction image (sixth measurement minus precontrast image) due to longer interval between measurements. Histology: Invasive ductal breast cancer recurrence with DCIS of the left breast ([14 mm] GII).

Increased Breast Cancer Risk

In industrialized countries, a woman's risk of being diagnosed with breast cancer during her lifetime is ~10%. A number of factors are known to increase this risk substantially (Table 11.**2**).

To date there are no studies substantiating the value of dynamic MR mammography for women with an increased risk of developing breast cancer. One should therefore consider all the more critically the recommendation of some groups to use MR mammography for the examination of young women with a family history of breast cancer, based upon the limited value of x-ray mammography due to the expected high parenchymal density. Our own experience warrants a caution against such an indication: Focal enhancement areas are found in over 30% of young women (e.g., myxoid fibroadenomas, intraindividual fluctuations). These occasionally require further diagnostic measures to rule out malignancy, including "unnecessary" open biopsy. Impressive corroborating data have been presented by Kuhl et al.. (1999). On the other hand, the incidence of breast cancer in women under 30 years of age is 0.07/1000 women (under 40 years of age, 1/1000). It follows that MR mammography performed for this indication leads to a large number of unnecessary open biopsies, while the probability of detecting an otherwise occult carcinoma is extremely low.

It is a different matter for women with a proven genetic alteration increasing the disposition for developing breast cancer (positive test for mutations in suppressor genes *BRCA1* and/or *BRCA2*). The risk of

Table 11.**2** Risk Factors for the Development of Breast Cancer (Lynch)

	Low Risk	High Risk	Relative Risk
Age	Young	Old	>4
Breast cancer in mother and sister	No	Yes	>4
Breast cancer in first-degree relative	No	Yes	2–4
First pregnancy	<20 years	>30 years	2–4
Personal history of breast cancer	No	Yes	2–4

developing breast cancer is much greater for these women and increases with increasing age to ~70% for 70-year-olds. Initial studies on women over the age of 30 years with mutations of a *BRCA* gene show that MR mammography performed yearly is highly sensitive for the detection of breast cancer (10 carcinomas/135 patients) and much superior to other imaging techniques (Kuhl et al. 1999).

> **Indication for MR mammography:**
> **Monitoring of high-risk patients**
> (***BRCA* mutations)**
>
> Initial studies indicate that MR mammography performed yearly greatly increases the sensitivity of detecting breast cancer in patients with a BRCA mutation.

12 Differential Diagnoses and Strategic Considerations

Focal Enhancement

Round or Ovoid, Homogeneously Enhancing Lesion with Well-defined Borders

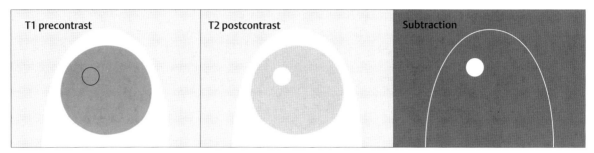

Fig. 12.**1**   Round or ovoid, homogeneously enhancing lesion with well-defined borders.

Differential diagnoses	
Common	**Rare**
Fibroadenoma (endotumoral septations), adenoma, papilloma, carcinoma (esp. NOS).	Intramammary lymph node (lipomatous hilus), fat necrosis (macrocalcification in mammogram), granuloma, carcinoma (esp. medullary form), phyllodes tumor, metastasis.

Differential diagnostic, i.e. therapeutic strategy (no corresponding finding in ultrasonography and mammography)			
Ultrasound and mammography **No findings (Bi-rads™1)**	**MR score** 0–3	**Size** All	**Consequence** None
	4	5–10 mm	Follow-up[1]
	4	> 10 mm	Excision

[1] Follow-up with MR mammography at six months interval.

Differential diagnostic, i.e. therapeutic strategy (with corresponding finding in ultrasonography and/or mammography)			
Ultrasound and mammography	**MR score**	**Size**	**Consequence**
Definitely benign (Bi-rads™2	0–3	All	None
	4	>5 mm	Excision
Probably benign (Bi-rads™3	0–2	All	None
	3	≦ 10	Follow-up[2]
	3	>10 mm	Needle biopsy[3]
	4	>5 mm	Excision
Possibly malignant (Bi-rads™4)	0, 1	All	None
	2–4	All	Excision
Highly suggestive of malignancy (Bi-rads™5)	0–4	All	Excision

[1] Follow-up with MR mammography at six months interval.
[2] Follow-up with ultrasound and/or mammography at six months interval.
[3] Ultrasound-guided or stereotactically guided needle biopsy.

Multiple Round or Ovoid, Homogeneously Enhancing Lesions with Well-defined Borders

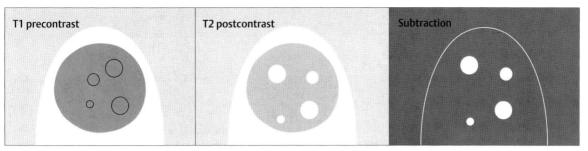

Fig. 12.**2** **Multiple round or ovoid, homogeneously enhancing lesions with well-defined borders.**

Differential diagnoses	
Common	**Rare**
Fibrocystic changes, fibroadenoma, adenoma, papilloma.	Multicentric carcinoma, metastases.

Differential diagnostic, i.e. therapeutic strategy (no corresponding finding in ultrasonography and mammography)			
Ultrasound and mammography	MR score[1]	Size	Consequence
No findings (Bi-rads™1)	0–3	All	None
	4	5–10 mm	Follow-up[2]
	4	>10 mm	Percutaneous biopsy/excision[3]

[1] Evaluation of 2–3 lesions.
[2] Follow-up with MR mammography at six months interval.
[3] MR-guided.

Differential diagnostic, i.e. therapeutic strategy (with corresponding finding in ultrasonography and/or mammography)			
Ultrasound and mammography	MR score[1]	Size	Consequence
Definitely benign (Bi-rads™2)	0–3	All	None
	4	>5 mm	Follow-up[2]
Probably benign (Bi-rads™3)	0–2	All	None
	3	≤10 mm	Follow-up[3]
	3	>10 mm	Needle biopsy[4]
	4	>5 mm	Excision
Possibly malignant (Bi-rads™4)	0, 1	All	None
	2–4	All	Excision
Highly suggestive of malignancy (Bi-rads™5)	0–4	All	Excision

[1] Evaluation of 2–3 lesions.
[2] Follow-up with MR mammography at 6 months interval.
[3] Follow-up with ultrasound and/or mammography at six months interval.
[4] Ultrasound-guided or stereotactically guided needle biopsy.

Round or Ovoid, Homogeneously Enhancing Lesion with Ill-defined Borders

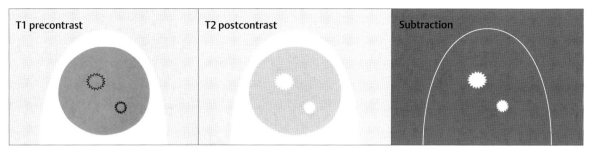

Fig. 12.**3**   **Round or ovoid, homogeneously enhancing lesion with ill-defined borders.**

Differential diagnoses	
Common	**Rare**
Fibrocystic changes, (sclerosing) adenosis, carcinoma.	Fat necrosis (history!), radial scar, DCIS, mastitis.

Differential diagnostic, i.e. therapeutic strategy (no corresponding finding in ultrasonography and mammography)			
Ultrasound and mammography	**MR score**	**Size**	**Consequence**
No findings (Bi-rads™1)	1–3	All	None
	4	5–10 mm	Follow-up[1]
	4	>10 mm	Percutaneous biopsy[2]
	5	>5 mm	Excision[3]

[1] Follow-up with MR mammography at six months interval.
[2] MR-guided.
[3] After MR-guided localization.

Differential diagnostic, i.e. therapeutic strategy (with corresponding finding in ultrasonography and/or mammography)			
Ultrasound and mammography	**MR score**	**Size**	**Consequence**
Definitely benign (Bi-rads™2)	1–3	All	None
	5	>5 mm	Excision
Probably benign (Bi-rads™3)	1–3	All	None
	4	≙_10 mm	Follow-up[1]
	4	>10 mm	Needle biopsy[2]
	5	>5 mm	Excision
Possibly malignant (Bi-rads™4)	1, 2	All	None
	3	All	Follow-up[3]
	4, 5	All	Excision
Highly suggestive of malignancy (Bi-rads™5)	1–5	All	Excision

[1] Follow-up with MR mammography at six months interval.
[2] Ultrasound-guided or stereotactically guided needle biopsy.
[3] Follow-up with ultrasound and/or mammography at six months interval.

Linear Contrast Enhancement

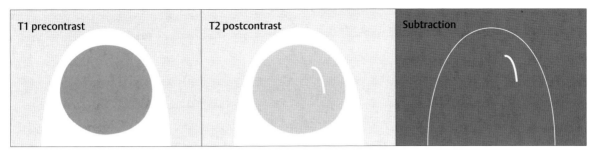

Fig. 12.**4**   **Linear contrast enhancement.**

Differential diagnoses	
Common	**Rare**
Motion artifacts in subtraction image (evaluation of single slices), intramammary veins.	DCIS, *Morbus Mondor* (superficial thrombophlebitis).

Differential diagnostic, i.e. therapeutic strategy (no corresponding finding in ultrasonography and mammography)			
Ultrasound and mammography	**MR score**	**Size**	**Consequence**
No findings (Bi-rads™1)	0–4	All	None
	5	>5 mm	Follow-up[1]

[1] Follow-up with MR mammography at six months interval.

Differential diagnostic, i.e. therapeutic strategy (with corresponding finding in ultrasonography and/or mammography)			
Ultrasound and mammography	**MR score**	**Size**	**Consequence**
Definitely benign (Bi-rads™2)	0–4	All	None
	5	>5 mm	Follow-up[1]
Probably benign (Bi-rads™3)	1–4	>5 mm	None
	5	>5 mm	Follow-up[1]
Possibly malignant (microcalcifications!) (Bi-rads™4)	0–5	All	Excision
Highly suggestive of malignancy (Bi-rads™5)	0–5	All	Excision

[1] Follow-up with ultrasound and/or mammography at six months interval.

Dendritic Contrast Enhancement

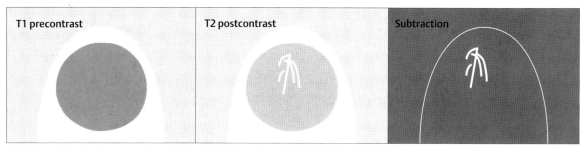

Fig. 12.**5** **Dendritic contrast enhancement.**

Differential diagnoses	
Common	**Rare**
Adenosis, fibrocystic changes, DCIS, motion artifacts in subtraction image (evaluation of single slices), superposition of intramammary veins.	Previous galactography (history), chronic mastitis.

Differential diagnostic, i.e. therapeutic strategy
(no corresponding finding in ultrasonography and mammography)

Ultrasound and mammography:	MR score	Size	Consequence
No findings (Bi-rads™1)	1–3	All	None
	4	>5 mm	Follow-up[1]
	5, 6	>5 mm	Excision[2]

[1] Follow-up with MR mammography at six months interval.
[2] After MR guided localization.

Differential diagnostic, i.e. therapeutic strategy
(with corresponding finding in ultrasonography and/or mammography)

Ultrasound and mammography	MR score	Size	Consequence
Definitely benign (Bi-rads™2)	1–4	All	None
	5, 6	>5 mm	Follow-up[1]
Probably benign (Bi-rads™3)	1–4	All	None
	5, 6	>5 mm	Follow-up[1]
Possibly malignant (microcalcifications!) (Bi-rads™4)	1–6	All	Excision
Highly suggestive of malignancy (Bi-rads™5)	1–6	All	Excision

[1] Follow-up with ultrasound and/or mammography at 6 months interval.

Spiculated Contrast-Enhancing Lesion

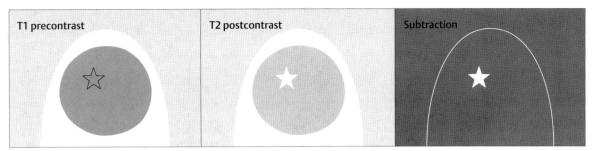

Fig. 12.**6**   **Spiculated contrast-enhancing lesion.**

Differential diagnoses	
Common	**Rare**
Fibrocystic changes, (sclerosing) adenosis, carcinoma.	Radial scar, carcinoma in scar tissue (history), DCIS, mastitis.

Differential diagnostic, i.e. therapeutic strategy (no corresponding finding in ultrasonography and mammography)			
Ultrasound and mammography	**MR score**	**Size**	**Consequence**
No findings (Bi-rads™1)	1–3	All	None
	4–8	<5 mm	Follow-up[1]
	4–8	>5 mm	Excision[2]

[1] Follow-up with MR mammography at six months interval.
[2] After MR-guided localization.

Differential diagnostic, i.e. therapeutic strategy (with corresponding finding in ultrasonography and/or mammography)			
Ultrasound and mammography	**MR score**	**Size**	**Consequence**
Definitely benign (Bi-rads™2)	1–3	All	None
	4–8	>5 mm	Excision
Probably benign (Bi-rads™3)	1, 2	All	None
	3	<10 mm	Follow-up[1]
	3	>10 mm	Needle biopsy[2]
	4–8	>5 mm	Excision
Possibly malignant (microcalcifications!) (Bi-rads™4)	1	All	None
	2–8	All	Excision
Highly suggestive of malignancy (Bi-rads™5)	1–8	All	Excision

[1] Follow-up with ultrasound and/or mammography at six months interval.
[2] Ultrasound-guided or stereotactically guided needle biopsy.

Lesion with Ring, i.e., Peripheral Enhancement

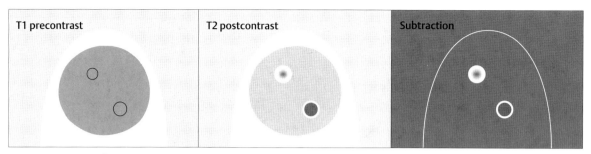

Fig. 12.**7** **Lesion with ring, i.e., peripheral enhancement.**

Differential diagnoses	
Common	**Rare**
Complicated cyst: narrow ring (cyst wall), hyperintense in T2-WI.	Adenosis, abscess, lymphadenitis.
Invasive carcinoma: broad ring (vital tumor), hypointense/isointense in T2-WI.	
Superposition of blood vessels (tubular structures in MIP image).	

Differential diagnostic, i.e. therapeutic strategy
(no corresponding finding in ultrasonography and mammography)

Ultrasound and mammography	MR score	Size	Consequence
No findings (Bi-rads™1)	2, 3	All	None
	>4	≤ 5 mm	Follow-up[1]
	>4	>5 mm	Excision[2]

[1] Follow-up with MR mammography at six months interval.
[2] After MR-guided localization.

Differential diagnostic, i.e. therapeutic strategy
(with corresponding finding in ultrasonography and/or mammography)

Ultrasound and mammography	MR score	Size	Consequence
Definitely benign (Bi-rads™2)	2, 3	All	None
	4–8	All	Excision
Probably benign (Bi-rads™3)	2	All	None
	3	<10 mm	Follow-up[1]
	3	>10 mm	Needle biopsy[2]
	4–8	>5 mm	Excision
Possibly malignant (Bi-rads™4)	2	All	None
	3–8	All	Excision
Highly suggestive of malignancy (Bi-rads™5)	2–8	All	Excision

[1] Follow-up with ultrasound and/or mammography at six months interval.
[2] Ultrasound-guided or stereotactically guided needle biopsy.

Diffuse Enhancement

Unilateral Diffuse Contrast Enhancement

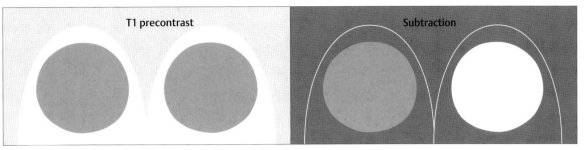

Fig. 12.**8**   **Unilateral diffuse contrast enhancement.**

Differential diagnoses	
Common	**Rare**
Parenchymal asymmetry, fibrocystic changes, adenosis, unilateral implant.	Normal finding (unfavorable cycle phase?, hormone replacement therapy?), mastitis, inflammatory breast cancer (clinical findings? skin changes?), extensive carcinoma (e.g. diffuse lobular carcinoma, lymphangiosis, extensive DCIS). Prior ipsilateral radiotherapy within the previous few months, prior contralateral radiotherapy several months before.

Differential diagnostic, i.e. therapeutic strategy
(no corresponding finding in ultrasonography and mammography)

Measurements in 2 to 3 representative areas are recommended. If strong initial contrast enhancement is present, MR mammography does not usually allow a reliable diagnostic evaluation. If applicable, repeat examination in favorable cycle phase or after terminating HRT: If findings are reproduced, (MR-guided) percutaneous biopsy is recommended. Otherwise no repeat examination should be performed.

Differential diagnostic, i.e. therapeutic strategy
(with corresponding finding in ultrasonography and/or mammography)

Ultrasound and/or mammography	Initial CE	Consequence
Definitely benign (Bi-rads™2)	Slight, moderate	None
	Strong	Follow-up[1]
Probably benign (Bi-rads™3)	Slight, moderate	None
	Strong	Needle biopsy
Possibly malignant (Bi-rads™4)	Slight, moderate, strong	Follow-up, needle biopsy, excision[2]
Highly suggestive of malignancy (Bi-rads™5)	Slight, moderate, strong	Needle, biopsy, excision[2]

[1] Follow-up with MR mammography at six months interval.
[2] Dependent upon clinical, mammographic, and/or ultrasonographic findings.

Bilateral Diffuse Contrast Enhancement

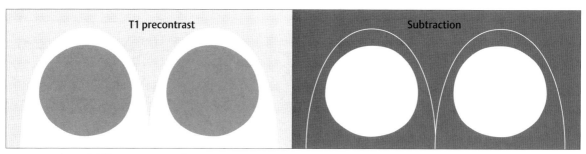

Fig. 12.**9** **Bilateral diffuse contrast enhancement.**

Differential diagnoses

Common	**Very rare**
Normal finding (unfavorable cycle phase?, hormone replacement therapy?), fibrocystic changes, adenosis.	Bilateral mastitis, bilateral inflammatory breast cancer (clinical findings? skin changes?), prior bilateral radiotherapy within the previous few months.

Differential diagnostic, i.e. therapeutic strategy
(no corresponding finding in ultrasonography and mammography)

Measurements in 2 to 3 representative areas are recommended. If strong initial contrast enhancement is present, MR mammography does not usually allow a reliable diagnostic evaluation. If applicable, repeat examination in favorable cycle phase or after terminating HRT. Otherwise no repeat examination should be performed. Thus there are no diagnostic or therapeutic consequences resulting from a MR mammography examination.

Differential diagnostic, i.e. therapeutic strategy
(with corresponding finding in ultrasonography and/or mammography)

Ultrasound and/or mammography	**Initial CE**	**Consequence**
Definitely benign (Bi-rads™2)	Slight, moderate, strong	None
Probably benign (Bi-rads™3)	Slight, moderate, strong	None
Possibly malignant (Bi-rads™4)	Slight, moderate, strong	Follow-up, biopsy, excision[1]
Highly suggestive of malignancy (Bi-rads™5)	Slight, moderate, strong	Biopsy, excision[1]

[1] Dependent upon clinical, mammographic, and/or ultrasonographic findings.

Table 12.**1**   Endotumoral and Peritumoral Changes

Endotumoral Changes	Differential Diagnosis	Peritumoral Changes	Differential Diagnosis
Calcification	• Fibroadenoma with macrocalcifications • Fat necrosis	Air	• Prior cyst aspiration/percutaneous biopsy
Fat	• Intramammary lymph node • Hamartoma • Oil cyst	Susceptibility artifacts	• Abscess (rare) • Prior open biopsy • Foreign body (e.g. needle)
Septations	• Fibroadenoma • Complicated cyst		• Breast expander • Subcutaneous port-a-cath
Fluid	• Cyst/complicated cyst • Ductectasia • Phyllodes tumor • Carcinoma • Abscess		• Sternal cerclage after thoracotomy • Piercing
Blood	• Hematoma • Complicated cyst • Prior percutaneous biopsy • Angiosarcoma		

13 Prosthesis Diagnostics

Examination Technique

Examinations performed for the purpose of detecting prosthesis complications are fundamentally different from those performed to rule out malignancy. First, no dynamic study is performed in such an examination, dispensing with the need for contrast administration. Second, special sequences are employed that allow the evaluation of the different prosthesis components (silicone, saline).

Measurement Protocols

The relative resonant frequencies of fat and silicone differ only slightly. Silicone has a resonant frequency ~100 Hz lower than that of fat, and ~320 Hz lower than that of water (Fig. 13.**1**). The most effective sequences for differentiating the different fluid components of a prosthesis are the inversion recovery (IR) sequences, which suppress the signal of fat. Using such IR sequences with an additional suppression of the water signal allows a signal-intense depiction of silicone, suppressing the signal of the saline component and surrounding fat tissue. On the other hand, IR sequences performed with the additional suppression of the silicone signal allow the selective depiction of the saline component. It is thus possible to separately image both prosthesis lumina of a double-lumen implant (silicone/water) in this way (Fig. 13.**2**).

Other measurement sequences used for the imaging of breast prostheses include fast SE sequences, with and

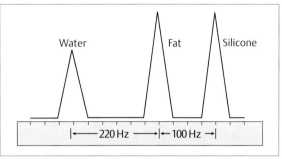

Fig. 13.**1**   **Resonant frequencies of fat, water, and silicone at 1.5 T.**

without water signal suppression. These sequences, however, do not allow such selective imaging of the prosthesis silicone component as can be achieved with the IR sequences described above.

In contrast to dynamic MR mammography, it is imperative for the examination of breast prostheses to use several angulations. Experience has shown the use of the sagittal slice orientation in addition to the usual axial slice orientation to be advantageous in imaging intramammary silicone cranially and caudally to the prosthesis, as well as deformation of the prosthesis in the cranio-caudal direction.

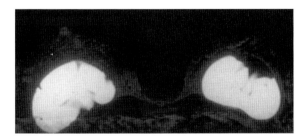
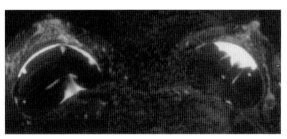

Fig. 13.**2 a,   b Water-sensitive   and   silicone-sensitive sequences.** Normal double-lumen prosthesis (saline/silicone).
a IR sequence with additional suppression of the water signal. Signal-intense imaging of the silicone component.

b IR sequence with additional suppression of the silicone signal. Signal-intense imaging of the saline component.

Normal Findings

Breast prostheses can be surgically implanted ventral to the pectoralis major muscle (**prepectoral position**) or dorsal to it (**subpectoral position**) (Figs. 13.**3** and 13.**4**).

The breast implant is typically oval in shape, or very rarely round. Deformation of the surface is not a pathological finding as long as the outer shell is intact (Fig. 13.**5**). The coating covering the implant may be smooth or textured. The shell of the implant is usually made of silicone elastomers and typically causes formation of a thin surrounding fibrous capsule after surgical implantation. Silicone found outside this capsule is pathological.

Due to the limited scope of this atlas, it is not possible to give detailed information on the great variety of silicone implants available on the market; for such information the reader is referred to specific literature. The following discourse is therefore confined to the materials most often used: saline and silicone.

When evaluating the internal structures of an implant, it is necessary to differentiate between single-lumen and double-lumen implants. The **single-lumen** prosthesis consists of a single chamber typically filled with a viscous silicone gel or (increasingly) saline. The **double-lumen** prosthesis consists of an inner chamber typically filled with a viscous silicone gel, and an outer chamber containing saline. A modification of this prosthesis in which the inner compartment contains saline and the outer compartment contains silicone is referred to as a "reverse double-lumen".

Folds of the outer shell into the lumen of the prosthesis (*radial folds*) are commonly seen. They are often only 1–2 cm long and represent a normal finding as long as they demonstrate a junction with the outer shell (Fig. 13.**6**).

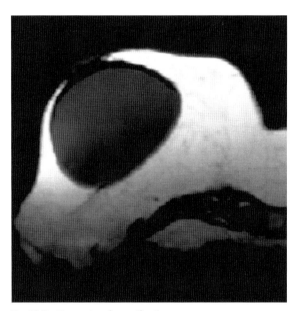

Fig. 13.**3** **Prepectoral prosthesis.**
Axial image of a single-lumen intramammary prosthesis.

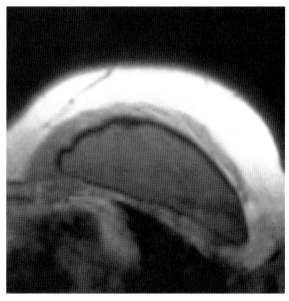

Fig. 13.**4** **Subpectoral prosthesis.**
Axial image of a prosthesis implanted dorsally to the pectoralis major muscle.

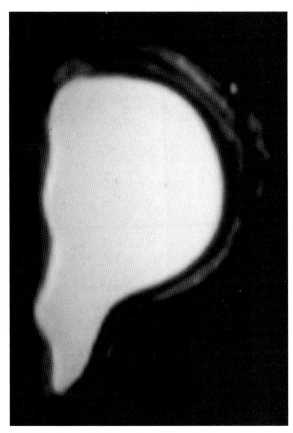

Fig. 13.**5   Normal deformation of prosthesis.**
MR image in sagittal slice orientation demonstrates nose-shaped protrusion of caudal portion of prosthesis.

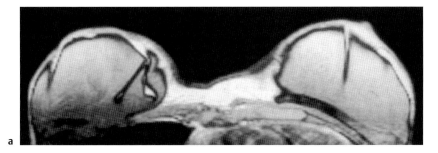

a

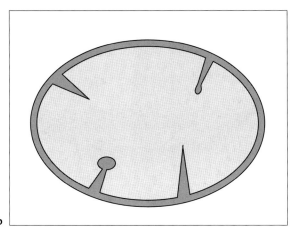

b

Fig. 13.**6 a, b   Radial folds.**
Short and long folds extending from the periphery into the lumina of both prostheses.

Complications

Capsular Contracture

Definition: Formation of a tough fibrous capsule around the prosthesis, which leads to pain and an undesirable deformation (contracture) of the implant. Extensive periprosthetic calcifications are often combined with these findings.

Classification of capsular contraction (according to Baker):

Grade I: Soft breast. Normal shape.
Grade II: Firm breast. Normal shape.
Grade III: Firm breast. Visible distortion.
Grade IV: Hard, painful breast. Marked spherical distortion.

Cave: Formation of a soft, nonpalpable periprosthetic capsule is a normal finding. Formation of a hard, thick fibrous capsule is pathological.

┌─ **General information**
│
│   **Incidence:**   Up to 20 % of all prostheses.
└

 MR mammography: Capsular contracture

A thickened periprosthetic capsule may show an increased contrast enhancement as the expression of a granulomatous inflammatory process (Fig. 13.**7**). Signal-free periprosthetic zones correspond to macrocalcifications. Deformation of the implant with acquisition of a spherical configuration is possible.

Cave: MR findings have low specificity. Diagnosis can only be made in the context of the clinical and mammographic findings.

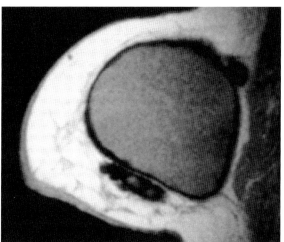
a

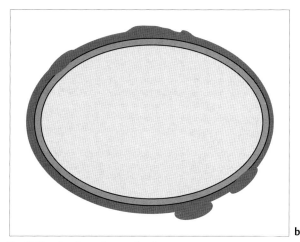
b

Fig. 13.**7 a, b   Capsular contracture.**
Thickening of the signal-free capsule. Additional signal-free periprosthetic areas correlate with extensive calcifications.

Silicone Bleed (Silicone Leaching)

Definition: Microscopic leakage of silicone out of the prosthesis through an intact implant shell. As a consequence, silicone accumulates between the fibrous capsule and the implant shell, i.e., within the radial folds (Fig. 13.**8**).

General information

Incidence:	No proven data. Most authors agree that all silicone gel implants bleed.

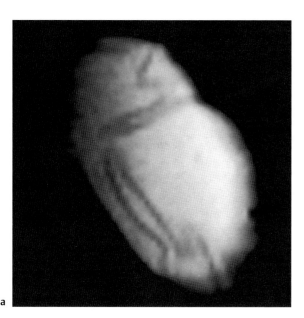

a

 MR mammography: "Teardrop" sign

Accumulation of silicone within the radial folds is most clearly visible at the keyhole-shaped terminal bend of the fold. A subtle analysis of these areas is therefore recommended.

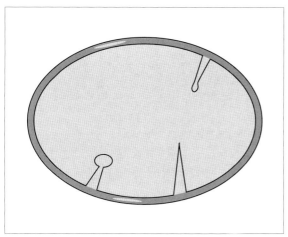

b

Fig. 13.**8 a, b   Silicone bleed.**
Silicone-equivalent signal within the radial folds, as well as between the capsule and implant shell as a sign of silicone bleed. Intact prosthesis capsule.

Intracapsular Rupture

Definition: Rupture of the implant shell, which typically collapses and then swims within the silicone gel. Released silicone lies outside the prosthesis but inside the intact fibrous capsule. Intracapsular ruptures occur in both single-lumen and double-lumen prostheses.
Cave: The term "intracapsular rupture" is not equivalent to a lesion of the internal of the two shells in a double-lumen prosthesis.

General information

| Incidence: | Approximately 80–90% of all prosthesis ruptures. |

 MR mammography: "Linguine sign"

Multiple curvilinear low-signal-intensity lines (corresponding to the collapsed prosthesis shell) are seen within the silicone-filled fibrous capsule. This is the most reliable indication of an intracapsular rupture. Silicone is not demonstrated outside the fibrous capsule (Figs. 13.**9** and 13.**10**).

Cave: Collapsed prosthesis shell versus radial fold.
Tip: Radial folds run from the periphery to the center. A collapsed prosthesis shell often runs parallel to the capsule.

"Salad-oil sign"
Drops of saline are seen floating within the silicone gel (Fig. 13.**11**). This is not a reliable sign of implant rupture. It can only be used as a diagnostic criterion indicating the presence of an intracapsular rupture in combination with the linguine sign.

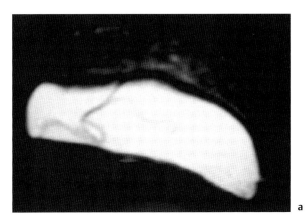

a

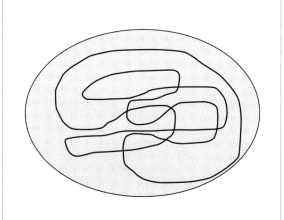

b

Fig. 13.**9 a, b   Intracapsular rupture.**
Collapsed prosthesis shell (linguine sign) within the fibrous capsule as proof of an intracapsular rupture. Surrounding capsule is intact.

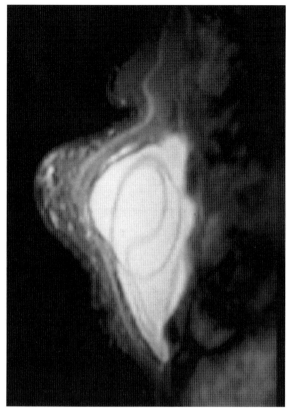
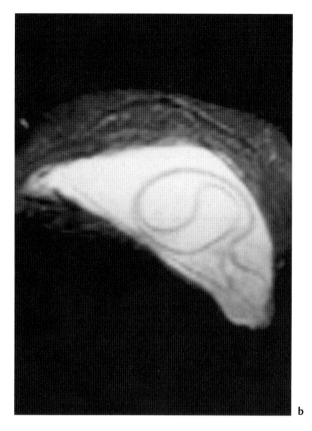

Fig. 13.**10 a, b   Intracapsular rupture.**
Intracapsular rupture with linguine sign. Single-lumen prosthesis.

a   Sagittal angulation.
b   Axial angulation.

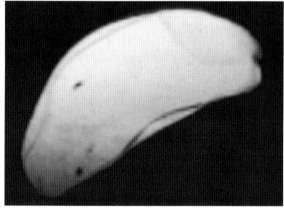
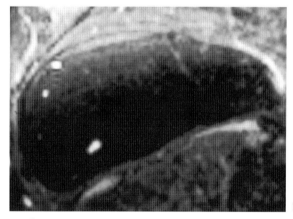

Fig. 13.**11 a, b   Intracapsular rupture.**
Intracapsular rupture with salad-oil-sign. Double-lumen prosthesis. Linguine sign was seen in cranial portions of the prosthesis (not shown).

a   Silicone-sensitive sequence.
b   Water-sensitive sequence.

Extracapsular Rupture

Definition: Rupture of both the implant shell and the fibrous capsule with macroscopic leakage of silicone into the surrounding tissues.

> **General information**
>
> **Incidence:**   Max. 20% of all prosthesis ruptures.

 MR mammography: Free silicone

Demonstration of silicone in the surrounding breast tissue outside the fibrous prosthesis capsule (Figs. 13.**12** and 13.**13**). An examination in at least two angulations is recommended to attain a complete depiction of all tissue closely surrounding the prosthesis. This is a definitive finding.

"Linguine sign"
The collapsed prosthesis shell seen within the silicone-filled fibrous capsule is a reliable indication of an intracapsular rupture. In combination with the demonstration of free silicone, it is often also seen in extracapsular ruptures.

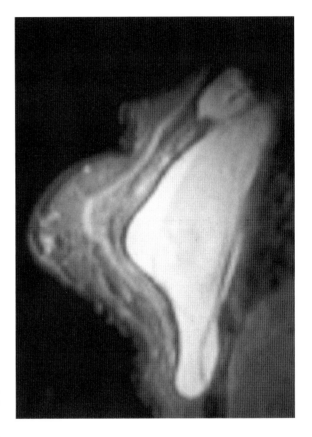

Fig. 13.**12   Extracapsular rupture.**   ▷
Extracapsular silicone ventral to the cranial portion of the prosthesis. Rupture of the implant shell (linguine sign) and surrounding fibrous capsule.

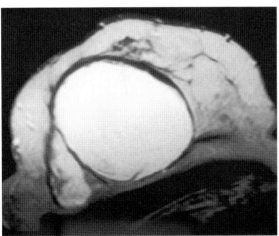

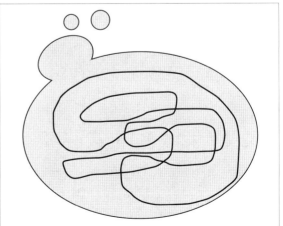

a   b

Fig. 13.**13 a, b   Extracapsular rupture.**
Free silicone outside the prosthesis capsule in the axillary tail of the breast.

Silicone Granuloma ("Siliconoma")

Definition: Collection of silicone within the breast parenchyma with concomitant granulomatous component, equivalent to a foreign-body granuloma. Occurrence after direct silicone injection into breast tissue or incomplete removal of a defective silicone prosthesis.

General information

Incidence:	Rare.

 MR mammography: Free silicone

Demonstration of focal areas of high signal intensity within the surrounding breast parenchyma is an indication of a localized collection of free silicone (silicone-sensitive sequence) (Fig. 13.**14**). Administration of contrast material is unnecessary. An examination in at least two angulations is recommended to attain a complete depiction of the silicone and determine its exact location.

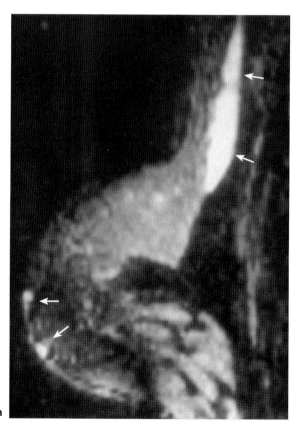

a

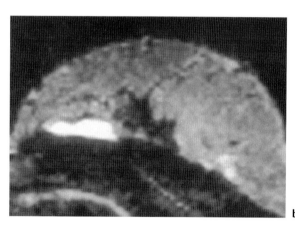

b

Fig. 13.**14 a, b Siliconoma.** Follow-up MRI examination after incomplete removal of a ruptured prosthesis.
a Silicone-sensitive sequence allows demonstration of signal-intense, oblong collections of silicone along the pectoral muscle and in the plane of the areola (arrows).
b Depiction of prepectoral silicone collection in examination with axial angulation.
Surgical excision of these siliconomas with histological confirmation.

Autologous Mammoplasty

Reconstructive surgery using tissue from a distant site is rarely performed in current breast surgery. In principle, different forms of tissue transposition surgery can be distinguished by MR mammography depending upon the tissue used. The most common techniques are the **latissimus dorsi myocutaneous flap** (Fig. 13.**15**), performed especially when the pectoralis muscle has been removed, and the **transverse rectus abdominis myocutaneous (TRAM) flap**, in which the supplying vascular bundle passes from the chest wall caudally (ipsilateral flap) or mediocaudally (contralateral flap) to the respective breast quadrant. Other types of myocutaneous flaps have also been described (e.g. contralateral upper rectus flap, vertical rectus flap).

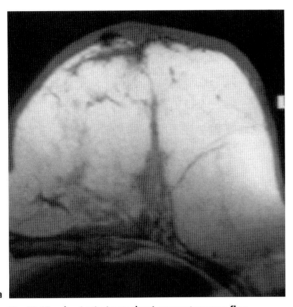
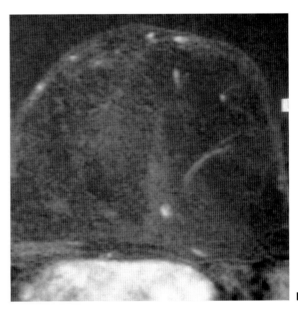

a

b

Fig. 13.**15 a, b   Latissimus dorsi myocutaneous flap.**

a T1-weighted GE sequence shows left breast composed of adipose tissue with central vascular bundle originating at the chest wall.

b Subtraction image with documentation of normal vascularization with discrete triangular enhancement within the non-lipomatous vascular bundle of the flap.

14 MR-guided Interventions

Indications for MR-guided Interventions

With the increasing use of dynamic MR mammography there is also an increasing number of cases in which MR mammographic findings suspicious of malignancy cannot be correlated to a clinical or conventional imaging finding. In such cases, and especially when the MR mammographic lesion is 1 cm in diameter or larger, the ultrasonographic examination should be repeated, paying special attention to exact location of the lesion. When the MR mammographic lesion is smaller than 1 cm in diameter, however, the chance of finding a correlating lesion in ultrasonography is relatively low.

There are three possible courses of action when a lesion has been identified by MR mammography only:

Ignore the lesion		**Not acceptable**
Follow-up (e.g., in 6 months)		**Acceptable** Note, however, that in the case of malignancy the diagnosis has been delayed for 6 months.
Further diagnostics		**Desirable** Specialized equipment is required.

Various groups have developed dedicated MR devices to perform percutaneous biopsies or preoperative localizations for the further evaluation of such lesions,.

MR-guided percutaneous biopsies can be performed as either a fine-needle aspiration biopsy or a large-core biopsy. It is recommended that only lesions of 10 mm in diameter or greater be biopsied in this way, since most systems do not reliably permit accurate biopsy of lesions with a smaller diameter.

MR-guided preoperative localization is performed to aid the surgeon in performing a well-aimed biopsy of the lesion while limiting the amount of excised tissue to a minimum. It also allows a rapid and selective examination of the biopsy material by the pathologist. In general, lesions of any size can be localized. It appears practical, however, to set a lower limit of 5 mm. The guidelines in Table 14.1 have proven useful as an orientation for the course of action to be taken in such cases.

Table 14.1 Course of Action in the Diagnostic Work-up of Suspicious MR Findings in the Breast

Lesion Size	MR Score	Course of Action
< 5 mm	< 4	No follow-up
	4–8	Follow-up in 6 months
5–10 mm	< 4	Follow-up in 6 months
	4–8	Open biopsy
> 10 mm	< 4	Percutaneous biopsy
	4–8	Open biopsy

Stereotactic Devices

The first attempts to perform MR-guided preoperative localizations used the so-called "free-handed technique" (Fischer et al. 1995; Sittek et al 1996). For this, cutaneous markers were positioned on the skin for orientation and the location of the lesion was estimated. Such methods were relatively inexact and should no longer be used given that stereotactic devices are now available.

A common characteristic of most devices for MR-guided interventions is the use of one or more perforated synthetic material plates for breast compression. After exact localization of a suspicious lesion, needles or localization wires can be inserted into the breast through the appropriate puncture channel. The various systems differ from one another, however, in the positioning of the patient (see Fig. 14.**3**).

The Göttingen Interventional Device

MR-guided breast interventions have been performed in our department since the end of 1993. For these, a dedicated device integrated into a customary commercial surface coil (so-called shoulder-flex coil, Siemens Co.), which allows the performance of interventions in the supine position, is used (Figs. 14.**1** and 14.**2**).

The puncture component consists of two semicircular hollow half-cylinders, which can be angled up to a maximum of 30° toward each other. This results in a better immobilization of the breast, and also allows the performance of interventions for abnormalities in the retromamillary region. Each of the semicircular components contains a total of 108 puncture channels arranged in parallel rows (two rows with 3 channels each, two rows with 5 channels each, four rows with 6 channels each, four rows with 7 channels each, and five rows with 8 channels each). The inner diameter of the channels (2.3 mm) allows the insertion of biopsy needles up to 14 gauge. The distance between the channels is 8 mm. Both hollow half-cylinders are filled with a 0.01 mol/l gadolinium solution. In the T1-weighted sequence the puncture channels are depicted as hypointense spaces within the surrounding signal intense solution.

The component described above is fixed to a commercial Plexiglas holding device. The use of this system with the patient in the supine position allows maximal freedom of movement and unlimited access to the breast, as well as a patient position identical to that under surgical conditions. The direct approach to the lesion in the compressed breast results in very short distances between the skin and the lesion, usually less than 3–4 cm, so that needle deviations are avoided. The major advantages of this system are the simple yet reliable handling, the low manufacturing costs due to the use of commercially available surface coils, and flexibility of use.

Biopsy Device (Halle)

In cooperation with the Siemens Co., Heywang-Köbrunner and co-workers developed a prototype of a circularly polarized, unilateral breast surface coil with integrated compression device. This system showed limitations in the biopsy of lesions near the chest wall (Heywang-Köbrunner et al. 1994). Later, this same group developed an aiming device (AD) that allowed the biopsy and localization of lesions outside the magnet tube (Heywang-Köbrunner et al. 1999).

With the patient in the prone position, the hanging breast is compressed and immobilized from the medial and lateral side by two plates, each consisting of several synthetic flexible ribs that can be spread apart to allow free access with any size of needle or other equipment. After imaging of the affected breast, the coordinates of the suspicious intramammary lesion are related to an externally defined so-called zero point. It is from this point that calculations for positioning (angulation and depth) the biopsy or localization needle are performed and the intervention is executed. Since positioning of the needle occurs outside the system, the correct placement of the needle cannot be imaged and verified. To date this device has mainly been used to perform percutaneous vacuum biopsies. The inability to document the topographic relationship between the localization wire tip and the suspicious lesion makes this system inadequate for use in MR-guided preoperative localizations (Fig. 14.**3a**).

Biopsy Device (Bonn)

Kuhl and colleagues have reported successful MR-guided biopsies and preoperative localizations using a localization and biopsy device from the Philips Co. The patient lies in a half lateral position with the breast immobilized by compression plates. Imaging is performed using a customary commercial circular ring coil placed under the breast (Kuhl et al. 1997). Needle biopsies are performed solely through the laterally placed plate. To date more than 300 patients have been examined using this system (Fig. 14.**3b**).

Biopsy Device (Leipzig)

Thiele and colleagues have reported MR-guided interventions using a GE Medical Systems open 0.5 T MRI unit. The intervention is performed with the patient in the sitting position using a bilateral breast biopsy holding fixture that immobilizes the breast with two compression plates. Imaging is accomplished using a flexible transmitting and receiving coil (Thiele et al. 1998) (Fig. 14.**3c**).

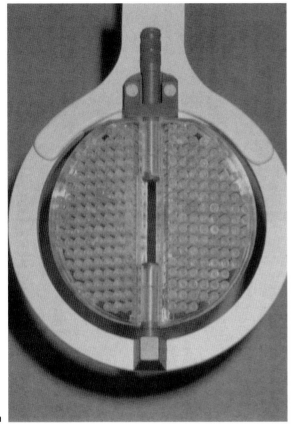

a

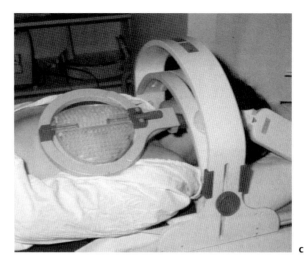

c

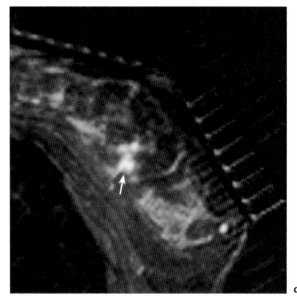

d

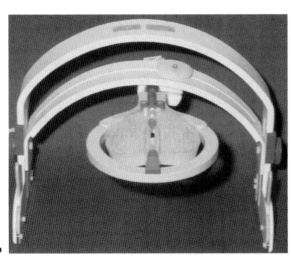

b

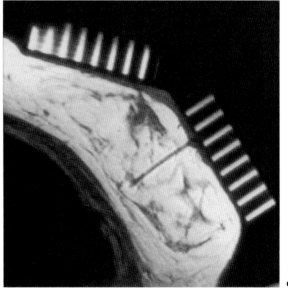

e

Fig. 14.**1 a–e** **The Göttingen interventional device.**
a View from above. Central puncture component and flex coil within the outer frame.
b Illustration of the complete system attached to a holding device.
c Demonstration of use with the patient in the supine position.
d Typical depiction in subtraction image. Documentation of a hypervascularized lesion (arrow).
e T1-weighted SE image with documentation of the needle after localization.

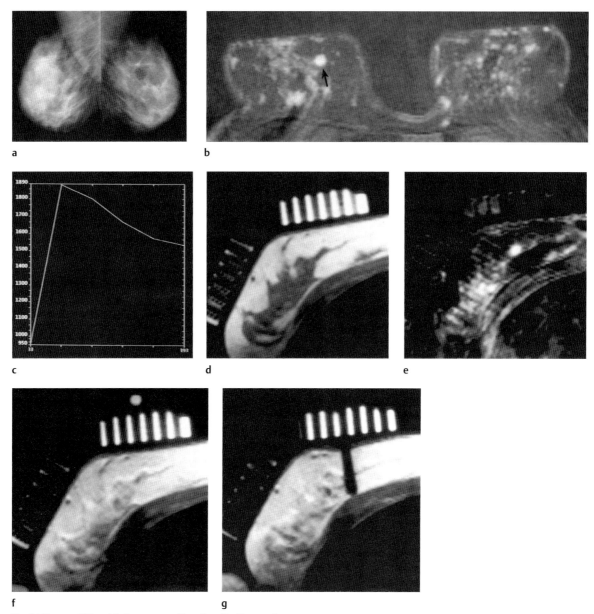

Fig. 14.**2 a–g MR-guided preoperative localization using the Göttingen interventional device.**
a Mammographically dense parenchyma.
b MR mammography (MIP technique) shows a suspicious lesion in the right breast (arrow).
c Signal analysis demonstrates a suspicious signal–time curve.

d MR-guided localization in a T1-weighted precontrast image.
e Demonstration of the lesion in subtraction image.
f Oil capsule marking of the channel intended for use.
g Verification of correct wire positioning in postlocalization MRI.
Histology: Invasive ductal carcinoma (pT1 GIII).

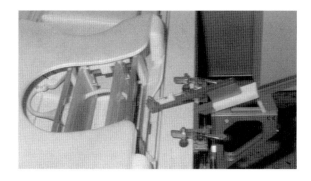
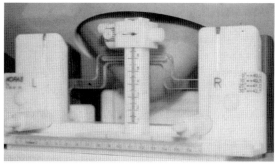
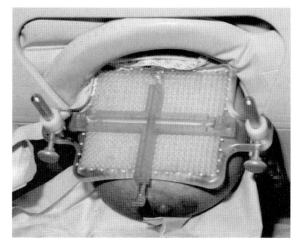
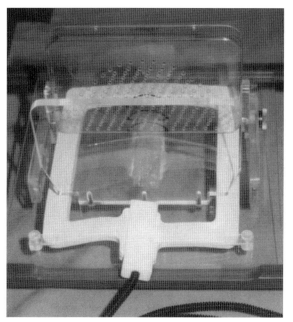
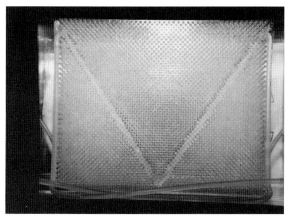

Fig. 14. **3 a–e   Various MR interventional devices.**
a Unilateral device of the University of Halle (Siemens Co.).
b Unilateral device of the University of Bonn (Philips Co.).
c Bilateral device (University of Leipzig).
d Bilateral device (University of Tübingen).
e Biopsy device of the Noras Co. (University of Leipzig).

Biopsy Device (Tübingen)

Müller-Schimpfle and colleagues have described a device permitting the bilateral biopsy of the breast (Müller-Schimpfle et al. 1998). Lateral compression plates were used with the patient in the prone position. For orientation—i.e., in order to identify the appropriate channel—an oil-filled M-shaped tube is integrated into the plate (Fig. 14.**3d**).

MR Breast Biopsy System

Noras Medizintechnik has presented a system for performing breast biopsies that can be added to the surface coil of the MRI Devices Corporation (Fig. 14.**3e**).

MRI-compatible Biopsy Equipment

The MR-guided percutaneous biopsy of the breast can be performed either as a fine-needle aspiration biopsy (22–18 gauge) (Table 14.**2**) or as a large-core biopsy (18–14 gauge) (Table 14.**3**). The industry provides a large number of different MRI-compatible materials for the performance of both of these methods (Fig. 14.**4**).

The listed fine-needle biopsy needles do not differ significantly in their extinction of the MR signal. Depending on the selected sequence, the degree of signal extinction (susceptibility artifact) caused by these needles lies between 5 mm (SE sequence) and 8 mm (GE sequence) (Fischer et al. 1997).

The listed large-core biopsy needles also do not differ significantly from one another in their extinction of the MR signal. Depending on the selected sequence, the degree of signal extinction (susceptibility artifact) caused by these needles lies between 7 mm (SE sequence) and 10 mm (GE sequence) (Fischer et al. 1997).

The major factors affecting the MR signal extinction are the selected sequence and the angulation of the needle in relation to the main magnetic field B_0. The signal extinction is least when the needle and the magnetic field are parallel. In comparison, the composition of the metal alloy (major components: titanium and nickel) makes no significant difference.

Suitable equipment is also available for performing large-core biopsies in coaxial technique (Table 14.**4**).

Table 14.**2**   MRI-compatible Fine-Needle Biopsy Needles (22–18 gauge)

Name	Manufacturer	Cut	Diameter (G)	Length (cm)
Lufkins' cytology needle	Guerbet	Chiba	22, 20, 18	5, 10, 15, 20
DAUM PunctureNeedle	Daum	Chiba	22, 20, 18	4, 5, 7.5, 10, 15
DAUM Aspiration BiopsyNeedle	Daum	Chiba	22, 18	7.5, 10, 15
MReye Chiba Biopsy Needle	Cook	Chiba	22, 19.5, 18	15, 20
MReye Franseen Lung Biopsy Needle	Cook	Franseen	22, 19.5, 18	15, 20
mrTool Chiba Nadel Ultra	Somatex	Chiba	21, 19.5, 18	9, 12, 15, 22, 28

Table 14.**3**   MRI-compatible Large-Core Biopsy Needles (18–4 gauge)

Name	Manufacturer	Diameter (G)	Length (cm)
MRI Biogun Large Core Biopsy Device	Guerbet	18, 14	10, 15
DAUM BiopsyNeedle	Daum	18, 14	7.5, 10, 15, 20
DAUM BiopsyGun	Daum	18, 16, 14	10, 15
MRT Biopsy Handy	Somatex	18, 16	10, 15, 20
mrTool Soma-Cut	Somatex	18, 14	6, 10, 15, 20

Table 14.**4**   MRI-compatible Coaxial Systems

Name	Manufacturer	Diameter (G)	Length (cm)
DAUM CoaxNeedle	Daum	for 20, 18, 16 G	10, 15, 20
mrTool coaxial needle	Somatex	for 0.8/1.2 mm	5, 10, 15

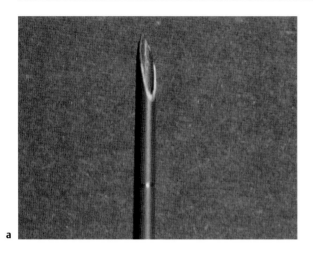

a

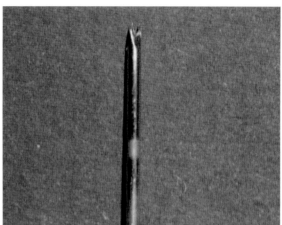

b

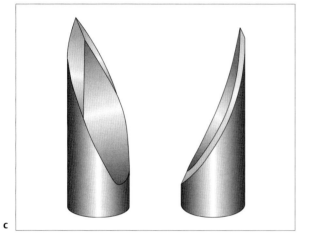

c

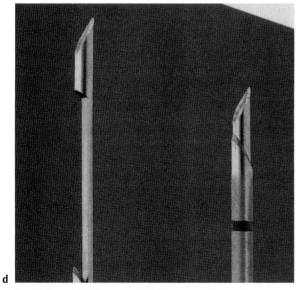

d

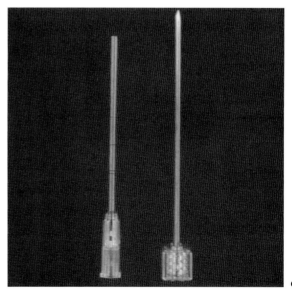

e

Fig. 14.**4 a–e   MRI-compatible biopsy equipment.**

a Fine-needle biopsy needle: Chiba cut (various manufacturers).

b Fine-needle biopsy needle: Franseen cut (e.g., Cook Co.).

c Biopsy cannula (Daum Co.) with SideSlit.

d Core cut biopsy cannula (various manufacturers).

e Coaxial system (various manufacturers).

MRI-compatible Localization Equipment

Various MR-compatible localization needles are available for the MR-guided preoperative localization of suspicious lesions (Fig. 14.5 and Tables 14.5–14.7). In terms of the wire configuration, they do not differ from the localization wires used for stereotactic and ultrasono-graphically guided localizations. However, the different types of localization wires are categorized into those whose position can be corrected and those that must be removed surgically after placement.

Table 14.**5** MRI-compatible Localization Material

Name	Manufacturer	Type	Diameter (G)	Length (cm)
Lesion localization system	Guerbet	Hook-wire	20	5, 7.5, 10
DuaLok MR	BARD	Double anchor[1]	??	7.7, 10.7
MReye Kopans Breast Lesion Localization Needle	Cook	Hook-wire	21, 20, 19	5, 9, 15
mrTool Localization Set	Somatex	Hook-wire	19.5, 18	5, 9, 12
mrTool Adjustable Localization Set	Somatex	U-formed[1]	20	5, 9, 12
DAUM LeLoc[T]	Daum	Hook-wire	18	5, 10, 15
DAUM LeLoc[T] D	Daum	Double hook	14	10
Marking-Coil	Cook	Ring	-	0.4

[1] Adjustment possible after misplacement.

The listed localization wires do not differ significantly in their extinction of the MR signal after removal of the conducting needle. Depending on the selected sequence, the degree of signal extinction (susceptibility artifact) caused by these wires lies between 3 mm (SE sequence) and 5 mm (GE sequence) (Fischer et al. 1997).

Another possibility for the preoperative localization of a MR lesion is the placement of a skin marker. This is acceptable provided that the lesion has a close topographic relation to a clearly reproducible skin structure (e.g., the nipple). Some groups favor the intramammary application of a gadolinium–charcoal suspension for preoperative localization of the lesion.

Table 14.**6** MRI-detectable Skin Markers

Name	Manufacturer	Diameter
CT-MRI Topographic Markers	E-Z-EM (Guerbet)	20 mm
Oil capsules (e.g. nitroglycerin)	Pohl	~ 5 mm

Table 14.**7** MRI-detectable Marker Suspension

1.4 ml charcoal suspension (4 g charcoal in 100 ml glucose solution)
+ 0.1 ml Gd solution (1 part 0.5 mmol Gd-DTPA/ml + 4 parts 5 % glucose solution)
Total volume = 1.5 ml (Heywang-Köbrunner 1995)

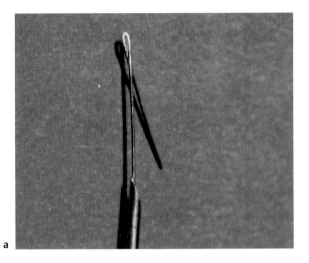

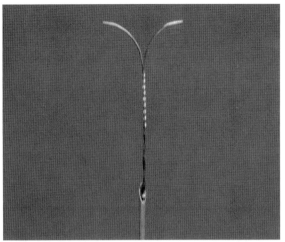

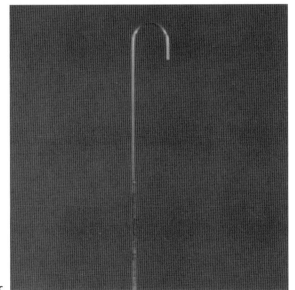

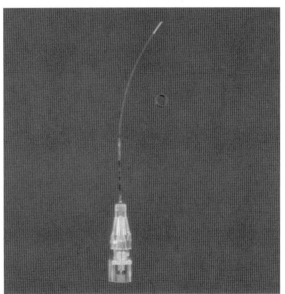

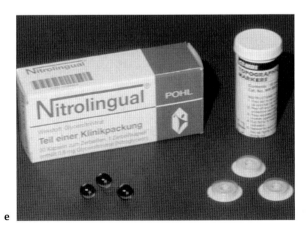

Fig. 14.**5 a–e MRI-compatible localization equipment.**
a Hook wire (various manufacturers).
b Double anchor (BARD Co.).
c U-shaped localization wire (Somatex Co.).
d Marking-Coil (Cook Co.).
e Skin markers (various manufacturers).

Confirmation of Complete Excision of Lesion

After the preoperative ultrasonographic or stereotactic localization of a suspicious lesion, the examination of the excised tissue in the perioperative setting with the appropriate technique allows confirmation of the complete removal of the lesion. Because the pathological tumor vascularization cannot be demonstrated with an imaging technique in excised tissue, however, it is not possible to confirm the removal of a lesion detected only by MR mammography.

Our studies with the intravenous administration of contrast medium a few minutes before surgical excision and subsequent MR imaging of the excised specimen did not produce satisfactory results. In addition, radiography of the specimen did not allow reliable identification of the respective lesion (Fischer et al. 1997).

As a consequence, it does not seem reasonable or possible at the present time to generally force an image representation of an MR-lesion within the excised specimen. It is, however, recommendable to perform a follow-up MR mammographic examination after the final histopathological diagnosis is obtained if this does not conform with the expected diagnosis. According to our experience, such an examination can be performed without difficulty up to 10 days after surgery. As is to be expected, postoperative changes such as hyperemia, seromas, and possibly hematomas are seen in these examinations. Nevertheless, since the size, position, and contrast enhancement characteristics of the localized suspicious lesion are known from the preoperative examination, it is usually possible to identify that a lesion has not been successfully excised in spite of the postoperative changes.

As an alternative, a follow-up MR mammographic examination can be performed for forensic reasons six months after surgery. Wound healing is complete after this period of time and the fibrotic scar tissue shows no disturbing contrast enhancement.

If the postoperative MR examination shows that, in spite of MR-guided preoperative localization of a suspicious lesion, it has not been fully removed, the patient must again undergo surgery for the excision of the lesion after repeat MR-guided localization (Fig. 14.**6**).

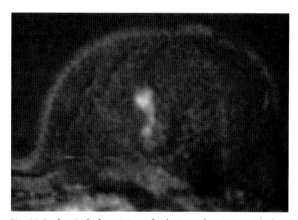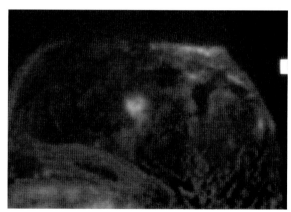

Fig. 14.**6 a,b   Failed excision of a lesion after MR-guided preoperative localization.**

a Dynamic MR mammography shows a lesion suspicious for malignancy with a satellite lesion.
Histology of excised specimen after preoperative MR-guided localization: Fibrocystic changes without epithelial proliferation.

b Follow-up MRI on the fifth postoperative day shows unchanged depiction of suspicious findings. Retromamillary seroma and diffuse contrast enhancement are seen as postoperative changes.
After repeat MR-guided localization, histology revealed confirmation of an invasive breast carcinoma.

Results

Several groups have reported MR-guided interventions of the breast in more or less large patient collectives. Primarily these interventions have been preoperative localizations. The number of published MR-guided biopsies to date is comparatively small.

Reports of the number of malignant findings ascertained by MR-guided **percutaneous biopsy** vary greatly (13–60%). On the one hand, this is due to the respective indications for biopsy; on the other, it depends on the type of equipment used (see Table 14.**8**).

Table 14.**8** MR-guided Percutaneous Biopsy

Group	City	Year	Number	Cytology/Histology Benign	Malignant	Failures
Fischer	Göttingen	1999	40	28 (70%)	9 (23%)	3
Heywang-Köbrunner	Halle	1997	31	23 (74%)	4 (13%)	2
Kuhl	Bonn	1997	10	0 (0%)	6 (60%)	4
Müller-Schimpfle	Tübingen	1999	8	6 (75%)	1 (13%)	1
Schmidt	Leipzig	1999	16	10 (63%)	5 (32%)	1
Sittek	Munich	1999	36	26 (72%)	10 (28%)	0

The results reported for MR-guided **preoperative localizations**, performed chiefly as wire localizations, are in substantial agreement. The average proportion of malignant tumors is ~50% (Table 14.**9**).

Table 14.**9** MR-guided Preoperative Localization

Group	City	Year	Number	Cytology/Histology Benign	Malignant
Fischer	Göttingen	1999	202	111 (55%)	91 (45%)
Heywang-Köbrunner	Halle	1997	27	15 (55%)	12 (45%)
Kuhl	Bonn	1997	110	44 (40%)	56 (56%)
Müller-Schimpfle	Tübingen	1999	31	18 (58%)	11 (36%)
Schmidt	Leipzig	1999	28	19 (68%)	9 (32%)
Sittek	Munich	1999	180	105 (58%)	75 (42%)

MR-guided vacuum core biopsy(Table 14.**10**) is presently considered "work in progress". It remains to be seen whether clear indications for this procedure can be defined that justify the greater effort required in comparison to a preoperative localization procedure.

Table 14.**10** MR-guided Vacuum Biopsy

Group	City	Year	Number	Cytology/Histology Benign	Malignant	Failures
Heywang-Köbrunner	Halle	1999	60	43 (72%)	16 (27%)	1

15 Quality Assessment

Check List for MR Mammography

Hardware

– System field strength 0.5–1.5 T?
– Bilateral breast surface coil?
– Breast compression device?
– MR-compatible biopsy equipment?

Software

– CM-sensitive sequence (T1-weighted GE sequence)?
– Correct echo time?
– Temporal resolution < 2 minutes/sequence?
– Spatial resolution ≤ 4 mm?
– No image overlap by phase-encoding gradient?

Appointment scheduling

– Correct indication?
– Adequate formulation of the diagnostic problem?
– Correct menstrual cycle phase?
– Oral hormonal therapy?
– Findings of other diagnostic procedures
  (clinical examination, mammography, ultrasonography)?
– Conventional mammogram in original?
– Former interventional diagnostic procedures
  (fine-needle biopsy, large-core biopsy, galactography)?
– Former therapeutic procedures
  (surgery, lumpectomy, radiotherapy)?

Image postprocessing

– Complete imaging of both breasts?
– Intramammary documentation of contrast material?
– Amount of motion artifacts is acceptable?
– Subtraction of corresponding precontrast from post-
  contrast images?
– Correct placement of ROI?

After recommendation of a follow-up MRI (six months)

– Reminder letter to patient who has failed to come in
  for examination

In case of open biopsy

– Feedback regarding histological results
– Necessity of postoperative follow-up MRI?

MR Mammography Report

The written dynamic MR mammography report should include a short reference to the results of previously performed diagnostic procedures, the diagnostic question to be answered, and other important relevant patient information. Following this comes information pertaining to the technique used, sequences performed, angulation, and amount and type of contrast material administered. A short account of the image postprocessing completes this segment of the report.

The descriptive portion of the report specifies the observed changes and pathology in the T1-weighted precontrast images and in the T2-weighted images (if performed). It is especially important to include here a description of the dynamic signal behavior after intravenous administration of contrast.

In the final assessment, the changes described are conclusively evaluated taking the clinical, ultrasonographic, and mammographic findings into account.

Note: Because the sensitivity of MR mammography for intraductal tumors is limited, the wording of the conclusion should state that "MR mammography shows no signs suggestive of invasive breast cancer" rather than "a malignant lesion can be excluded" when no hypervascularized areas are detected.

In conclusion, clear recommendations for further action should be made (e.g., "Follow-up MR mammography in six months", "Open biopsy is recommended to rule out malignancy").

 Example:
Contrast-enhanced MR mammography on 11. 11. 2011

Personal history
Clinical, mammographic, and ultrasonographic findings suggest a malignant lesion of 1 cm in the upper outer quadrant of the left breast. MR mammography was performed as part of local preoperative staging. No known risk factors for breast cancer.

Technique and findings
Examination in 2D-technique with axial slice orientation using a T1-weighted GE sequence was performed once before, and repetitively after administration of 0.1 mmol Gd-DTPA/kg BW. Additional generation of axial T2-weighted TSE images. Postprocessing with image subtraction (seconnd measurement post-CM minus precontrast image) and signal–time analysis in relevant ROI.

No remarkable findings in T1-weighted precontrast image and T2-weighted measurements. After intravenous contrast administration demarcation of a strongly enhancing, spiculated, partially ill-defined lesion of 1 cm diameter in the upper outer quadrant of the left breast (initial contrast enhancement = 120%, postinitial washout). In addition, oval, well-defined lesion of 8 mm diameter in the upper inner quadrant of the left breast (initial contrast enhancement = 110%, postinitial plateau, ring-enhancement). No remarkable findings in the right breast.

Conclusion
In accordance with clinical, mammographic, and ultrasonographic findings, documentation of a localized lesion with characteristics typical of malignancy in the upper outer quadrant of the left breast. Documentation of an additional lesion suspicious of malignancy in the upper inner quadrant of the left breast, suggesting multicentric tumor spread. Surgical excision of this second MR mammographic lesion should be performed in the course of the primary operative procedure after preoperative MR-guided localization. No pathological findings within the right breast.

MR Breast Phantom

In cooperation with Dr. W. Döler (Medical Physics Department, University of Göttingen), a phantom that allows the simulation of the most important aspects of contrast-enhanced MR mammography has been designed and constructed (Figs. 15.**1**–15.**3**). This phantom comprises four components, some of which can be removed as single elements and exchanged. The system is made of polyvinyl chloride and can be used in any surface coil (Fischer et al. 1999).

Component 1

A total of three rows of small tubes containing different concentrations of CM are arranged in the medial (two rows of seven tubes each) and lateral (one row of eight tubes) portions of this phantom component. The CM concentrations range from 8 mmol/l to 0.0062 mmol/l in ascending and descending dilutions.

- *Purpose*: To correlate the signal intensity with the CM concentrations as a function of the location within the surface coil.

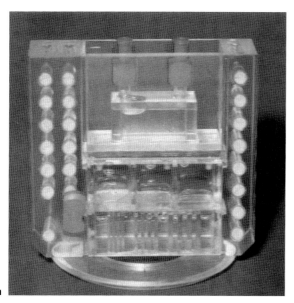

a

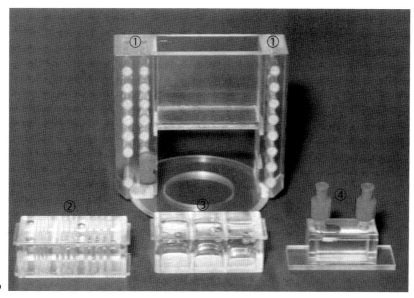

b

Fig. 15.**1 a, b   MR breast phantom.**
a Phantom in assembled state.
b Phantom elements in disassembled state. Single components numbered 1 to 4.

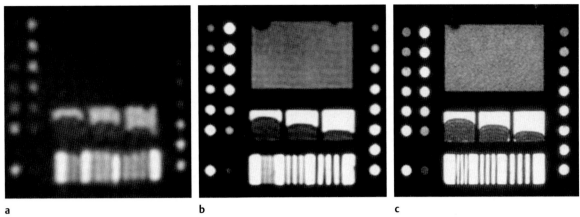

a

b

c

Fig. 15.**2 a–c Phantom studies using different sequences.**
Obvious differences in the quality of the phantom image depending on the sequence used.

a T1-weighted Turbo-FLASH sequence.
b T1-weighted FLASH sequence.
c T1-weighted SE sequence.

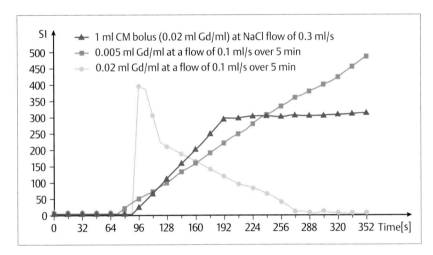

Fig. 15.**3 Simulation of signal–time curves.**
Simulation of three typical signal–time curves using the MR breast phantom.

Component 2

This component is a container measuring 6 cm × 2 cm × 3 cm. A total of 12 small synthetic plates with three different widths (four of 2 mm each, four of 1.5 mm each, four of 1 mm each) are set into this component with a distance of 1–2 mm separating them. The container is filled with a 0.5 mmol/l gadolinium solution.

• *Purpose*: To evaluate the spatial resolution.

Component 3

Three units, each 2 cm × 2 cm × 3 cm in size, contain a mixture of an oily fluid and water in different proportions (oil/water: 2/10, 6/6, 10/2).

• *Purpose*: To demonstrate in-phase or out-of-phase imaging.

Component 4

This dynamic mixing chamber (4 cm × 2 cm × 2 cm) has a feeding access and a draining access (Lüer connec-

tions). The feeding connection is used for mechanical injection (e.g., Spectris, Medrad Co.) of contrast solutions using commercially available infusion systems. The drainage of fluids from the second opening is also accomplished over an infusion system into a collection vessel.

• *Purpose*: To simulate different signal–time curves.

For quality assurance, the MR breast phantom allows comparison of existing sequences, optimization of measurement protocols, and verification of image constancy in routine practice. It can also serve as an illustrative aid in teaching. Additionally, it makes possible a direct comparison of different examination systems, and the specific adaptation of study protocols to such systems possible, e.g., for the realization of multicenter studies.

An MR breast phantom is commercially available from Nuclear Associates Co. It does not, however, allow the simulation of dynamic aspects of MR mammography.

16   Present Standing and Perspectives of MR Mammography

Present Standing

MR mammography is the method of choice in the diagnostic work-up of breast implant complications. The use of special sequence protocols, the selective imaging of the different prosthesis components, and the capability for multiplanar slice orientation make it superior to other breast imaging techniques.

In the diagnostic work-up for breast cancer, the clinical examination, x-ray mammography, and the percutaneous biopsy are of primary importance. Breast ultrasonography is a significant and useful complementary technique. While these methods all provide information about morphological changes in the breast, contrast-enhanced MR mammography primarily delivers information on vascularization and altered perfusion conditions within tumors.

Contrast-enhanced MR mammography has been proven to be the most sensitive technique in the detection of invasive breast cancer if the generally accepted indications for its performance are adhered to. Although the specificity is often considered to be too low, it is certainly acceptable and comparable to that of the other imaging techniques when it is used selectively and evaluated adequately. A technically perfect MR mammography examination that shows no contrast enhancement reliably rules out the presence of invasive breast cancer greater than ~5 mm in diameter.

The most important applications of MR mammography are local preoperative staging and follow-up examinations after breast-conserving therapy for breast cancer. This is confirmed by numerous reports from different groups. It is, none the less, often helpful and decisive in cases of uncertain constellations of findings in x-ray mammography and/or ultrasonography. In such cases, however, the diagnostic potential of all primary diagnostic techniques (clinical examination, x-ray mammography, percutaneous biopsy, and ultrasonography) should be fully exhausted before MR mammography, as the most costly of all techniques, is performed.

The uncritical performance of MR mammography must also be cautioned against because it can be presumed that this would lead to a significant increase in unnecessary open biopsies. As examples, a suspicious palpable abnormality or indeterminate microcalcifications on mammography do not constitute indications for the performance of MR mammography. This is also true for inflammatory changes. Apart from the performance of MR mammography in patients with a *BRCA* gene abnormality, there are no data suggesting advantages in performing this technique, for example, in young women with an increased risk factor for breast cancer.

In summary, MR mammography is an established and standardized examination method that increases the effectiveness of early breast cancer detection when used for defined indications as a complementary technique.

Perspectives

Further technical and methodological developments in MR mammography can be expected to be primarily in the improvement of spatial resolution (slice thickness from 1 to 2 mm). The incidental development of the examination protocols will yield an increasing amount of data, making efficient computers and user-friendly software necessary for rapid and standardized image postprocessing.

It remains to be seen whether new contrast materials will allow better differentiation of hypervascularized lesions in the breast. Possible examples are substances with a longer intravascular retention period ("blood-pool" agents). In the longer term, it is conceivable that tumor-specific contrast materials may become available.

A short-term expectation is that the importance of MR mammography as a diagnostic method of choice for women with a high genetic risk for breast cancer (*BRCA* gene mutations) will be substantiated in studies with larger patient collectives. This high-risk situation will then emerge as a further indication for the performance of MR mammography.

It can be assumed that the combination of a reduced radiation dose, single projection x-ray mammogram (e.g., full-field digital mammography in the MLO projection) with a contrast-enhanced MR mammography examination will have the highest sensitivity for the detection of breast cancer. Larger studies must examine whether such a diagnostic strategy is cost-effective for use in the screening of high-risk women. In this context, it is conceivable that dedicated diagnostic units specially designed for the MRI examination of the breast might be developed and produced for the breast cancer screening of this defined group of women. A high examination frequency using such dedicated, less expensive MRI units could significantly reduce the costs of MR mammography examination.

Most MR-guided breast interventions continue to be preoperative localizations of otherwise occult lesions. Examination units allowing "real-time-monitoring" have the advantage of decreased time expenditure; complex stereotactic equipment is therefore unnecessary. MRI-monitored interstitial laser photocoagulation, or complicated interventions such as MRI-guided minimally invasive diagnostic and therapeutic procedures, will remain limited to a few indications and will be performed in a handful of specialized centers.

References

History of MR Mammography, Patient preparation and information, Technique and Methods

Boetes CB, Barentsz JO, Mus RD et al. (1994). MR Characterization of Suspicious Breast Lesions with a Gadolinium-enhanced TurbFLASH Subtraction Technique. Radiology 193: 777–781

Buckley DL, Mussurakis S, Horsman A (1998). Effect of Temporal Resolution on the Diagnostic Efficacy of Contrast-Enhanced MRI in the Conservatively Treated Breast. JCAT 22: 47–51

Damadian R (1971). Tumor Detection by Nuclear Magnetic Resonance. Sciene 171: 1151–1153

Daniel BL, Butts K, Glover GH et al. (1998). Breast Cancer: Gadolinium-enhanced MR Imaging with a 0.5-T Open Imager and three-point Dixon Technique. Radiology 207: 183–190

El Yousef SJ, Alfidi RJ, Duchesneau RH (1983). Initial Experience with Nuclear Magnetic Resonance (NMR) Imaging of the Human Breast. J Assist Comput Tomogr 7: 215–218

Fischer U, von Heyden, Vosshenrich R et al. (1993). Signalverhalten maligner und benigner Läsionen in der dynamischen 2 D-MRT der Mamma. RÖFO 158: 287–292

Fischer U, Vosshenrich R, Kopka L et al. (1996). Kontrastmittelgestützte dynamische MR-Mammographie nach diagnostischen und therapeutischen Eingriffen der Mamma. Bildgebung 63: 94–100

Frahm, J, Haase A, Matthaei D (1986). Rapid Three-dimensional NMR Imaging Using the FLASH Technique. J Comput Assist Tomogr 10: 363–368

Haase, A, Frahm J, Matthaei D, et al. (1986). FLASH-Imaging: Rapid NMR Imaging Using Low Flip Angle Pulses. J Magn Res 67; 258–266

Harms SE, Flamig DP, Hesley KL et al. (1993). Fat-suppressed Three-dimensional MR Imaging of the Breast. Radiographics 1: 247–267

Heiberg EV, Perman WH, Herrmann VM, Janney CG (1996). Dynamic Sequential 3D Gadolinium-enhanced MRI of the Whole Breast. Magn Reson Imaging 14: 337–348

Heywang SH, Fenzl G, Beck R et al. (1986). Anwendung von Gd-DTPA bei der kernspintomographischen Untersuchung der Mamma. RÖFO 145: 565–571

Heywang SH, Fenzl G, Edmaier M, et al. (1985). Kernspintomographie in der Mammadiagnostik. RÖFO 143: 207–212

Heywang-Köbrunner SH, Haustein J, Pohl C et al. (1994). Contrast-enhanced MR Imaging of the Breast: Comparison of two Different Doses of Gadopentetate Dimeglumine. Radiology 191: 639–646

Heywang-Köbrunner SH, Beck R (1995). Contrast-enhanced MRI of the Breast. Springer-Verlag Berlin Heidelberg New York

Hulka CA, Smith BL, Sgroi DC et al. (1995). Benign and Malignant Breast Lesions: Differentiation with Echo-Planar MR Imaging. Radiology 197: 33–38

Kaiser WA, Zeitler E (1985). Kernspintomographie der Mamma – Erste klinische Ergebnisse. Röntgenpraxis 38: 256–262

Kaiser WA (1993). MR-Mammography (MRM). Springer-Verlag Berlin Heidelberg New York

Klengel S, Hietschold V, Schreiber M, Köhler K (1994). Quantitative kontrastmitteldynamische Mamma-MRT am 0.5-Tesla-Gerät. Röntgenpraxis 47: 223–228

Knopp MV, Port RE, Brix G et al. (1995). Diagnostische Wertigkeit der Quantifizierung der dynamischen Mammographie mit Hilfe pharmakokinetischer Parameter. Radiologe 35 (suppl): 84

Kuhl CK, Seibert C, Sommer T et al. (1995). Fokale und diffuse Läsionen in der dynamischen MR-Mammographie gesunder Probandinnen. RÖFO 163: 219–224

Kuhl CK, Kreft BP, Hauswirth A et al. (1995). MR-Mammographie bei 0.5 Tesla. Teil I: Vergleich von Bildqualität und Sensitivität der MR-Mammographie bei 0.5 und 1.5 T. RÖFO 162: 381–389

Kuhl CK, Kreft BP, Hauswirth A et al. (1995). MR-Mammographie bei 0.5 Tesla. Teil II: Differenzierbarkeit maligner und benigner Läsionen in der MR-Mammographie bei 0.5 und 1.5 T. RÖFO 162: 482–391

Kuhl CH, Bieling HB, Lutterberg G et al. (1996). Standardisierung und Beschleunigung der quantitativen Analyse dynamischer MR-Mammographien durch Parameterbilder und automatisierte ROI-Definition. Fortschr Röntgenstr 164: 475–482

Kuhl CH, Klaschik S, Mielcarek P et al. (1999). Do T2-weighted pulse Sequences help with the Differential Diagnosis of Enhancing Lesions in Dynamic Breast MRI? JMRI 9: 187–196

Laniado M, Kopp AF (1997). Gegenwärtiger Stand der klinischen Entwicklung von MR-Kontrastmitteln. RÖFO 167: 541–550

Lauterbur PC (1973). Image Formation by Induced Local Interactions: Examples Employing Nuclear Magnetic Resonance. Nature 242: 190–191

Magnevist Gadolinium-DTPA. Eine Monographie. Hrsg.: Felix R, Heshiki A, Hosten N, Hricak H. Blackwell Verlag 1997

Mansfield P, Morris PG, Ordidge R et al. (1979). Carcinoma of the Breast Imaged by Nuclear Magnetic Resonance (NMR). Brit J Radiol 52: 242–243

Mussurakis S, Buckley DL, Horsman A (1997). Dynamic MRI of Invasive Breast Cancer: Assessment of Three Region-of-Interest Analysis Methods. JCAT 21: 431–438

Müller-Schimpfle M, Rieber A, Kurz S et al. (1995). Dynamische 3D MR-Mammographie mit Hilfe einer schnellen Gradienten-Echo-Sequenz. RÖFO 162: 13–19

Müller-Schimpfle M, Ohmenhäuser K, Claussen CD (1997). Einfluß von Alter und Menstruationszyklus auf Mammographie und MR-Mammographie. Radiologe 37: 718–725

Niendorf HP, Haustein J, Cornelius I et al. (1991). Safety of Gadolinium-DTPA; Extended Clinical Experience. Magn Res Med 22: 222–228

Nunes LW, Schnall MD, Siegelman ES et al. (1997). Diagnostic Performance Characteristics of Architectural Features Revealed by High Spatial-Resolution MR Imaging of the Breast. AJR 169: 409–415

Perman WH, Heiberg EV, Herrmann VM (1996). Half-Fourier, Three-dimensional Technique for Dynamic Contrast-enhanced MR Imaging of Both Breasts and Axillae: Initial Characterization of Breast Lesions. Radiology 200: 263–269

Pierce WB, Harms SE, Flamig DP et al. (1991). Three-dimensional Gadolinium-enhanced MR Imaging of the Breast. Pulse Sequence with Fat Suppression an Magnetization Transfer Contrast. Radiology 181: 757–763

Ross RJ, Thompson JS, Kim K, Bailey RA (1982). Nuclear Magnetic Resonance Imaging and Evaluation of Human Breast Tissue: Preliminary Clinical Trials. Radiology 143: 195–205

Schmiedl U, Maravilla KR, Gerlach R, Dowling CA (1990). Excretion of Gadopentetate Dimeglumine in Human Breast Milk. AJR 154: 1305–1306

Schorn C, Fischer U, Döler W et al. (1996). Compression Device to Reduce Motion Artifacts at Contrast-enhanced MR Imaging in the Breast. Radiology 206: 279–282

Schorn C, Fischer U, Luftner-Nagel S, Grabbe E (1999). Diagnostic Potential of Ultrafast Contrast-Enhanced MRI of the Breast in Hypervascularized Lesions: Are there Advantages in Comparison with Standard Dynamic MRI? JCAT 23: 118–122

Teubner J, Behrens U, Walz M et al. (1995). Dynamische Visualisierung der Kontrastmittelaufnahme bei der Mamma-MRT. Radiologe 35 (suppl): 83

Weinmann HJ, Laniado M, Mützel W (1984). Pharmacokinetics of Gadolinium-DTPA/dimeglumine after Intravenous Injection into healthy Volunteers. Physiol Chem Phys Med NMR 16: 167–172

Weinmann HJ (1997). Eigenschaften von Gd-DTPA-Dimeglumin. In: Magnevist Gadolinium-DTPA. Eine Monographie. Hrsg.: Felix R, Heshiki A, Hosten N, Hricak H. Blackwell Verlag 1997

Weinstein D, Strano S, Cohen P et al. (1999). Breast Fibroadenoma: Mapping of Pathophysiologic Features with Three-Time-Point, Contrast-enhanced MR Imaging-Pilot Study. Radiology 210: 233–240

Wong TZ, Lateiner JS, Mahon TG et al. (1996). Stereoscopically Guided Characterization of Three-dimensional Dynamic MR Images of the Breast. Radiology 198: 288–291

Tumor Angiogenesis

Aranda FI, Laforga JB (1996). Microvessel Quantification in Breast Ductal Invasive Carcinoma. Correlation with Proliferative Activity, Hormonal Receptors and Lymph Node Metastases. Pathol Res Pract 192: 124–129

Bicknell-R; Harris-AL (1996). Mechanisms and Therapeutic Implications of Angiogenesis. Curr Opin Oncol 8: 60–5

Brinck U, Fischer U, Korabiowska M et al. (1995). The Variability of Fibroadenoma in Contrast-enhanced Dynamic MR-Mammography: AJR 168: 1331–1334

Buadu LD, Murakami J, Murayama S et al. (1997). Patterns of Peripheral Enhancement in Breast Masses: Correlation of Findings on Contrast Medium Enhanced MRI with Histologic Features and Tumor Angiogenesis. JCAT 21: 421–430

Buadu LD, Murakami J, Murayama S et al. (1996). Breast Lesions: Correlation of Contrast Medium Enhancement Patterns on MR Images with Histopathologic Findings and Tumor Angiogenesis. Radiology 200: 639–649

Buckley, DL, Drew PJ, Mussurakis S et al. (1997). Microvessel Density of Invasive Breast Cancer assessed by Dynamic Gd-DTPA enhanced MRI. J Magn Reson Imaging 7:461–464

Costello P, McCann A, Carney DN, Dervan PA (1996). Prognostic Significance of Microvessel Density in Lymph Node Negative Breast Carcinoma. Hum Pathol 26: 1181–1184

Engels K, Fox SB (1997). Angiogenesis as a Biologic and Prognostic Indicator in Human Breast Carcinoma. EXS 79: 113–156

Fischer U (1998). Aktuelle Aspekte der dynamischen MR-Mammographie. Habilitationsschrift Universität Göttingen

Folkman J, Klagsbrunn M (1987). Angiogentic Factors. Science 235: 442

Folkman J (1995). Clinical Applications of Research on Angiogenesis. N Engl J Med 333: 1757–1763

Frouge C, Guinebretiere JM, Contesso G et al. (1994). Correlation between Contrast Enhancement in Dynamic Magnetic Resonance Imaging of the Breast and Tumor Angiogenesis. Invest Radiol. 29: 1043–1049

Furman-Haran E, Margalit R, Maretzek AF, Egani H (1996). Angiogenic Response of MCF7 Human Breast Cancer to Hormonal Treatment: Assessment by dynamic Gd-DTPA-enhanced MRI at high Spatial Resolution. J Magn Reson Imaging 6:195–202

Goulding H, Rashid NA, Robertson JF et al. (1996). Assessment of Angiogenesis in Breast Carcinoma: An Important Factor in Prognosis. Hum Pathol 26: 1196–1200

Gradishar WJ (1997). An Overview of Clinical Trials Involving Inhibitors of Angiogenesis and their Mechanism of Action. Invest New Drugs 15: 49–59

Hulka CA, Edmister WB, Smith BL et al. (1997). Dynamic Echo-Planar Imaging of the Breast: Experience in Diagnosing Breast Carcinoma and Correlation with Tumor Angiogenesis. Radiology 205: 837–842

Paku S (1998). Current Concepts of Tumor-induced Angiogenesis. Pathol Oncol Res. 4: 62–75

Pluda JM (1997). Tumor-associated Angiogenesis: Mechanisms, Clinical Implications, and Therapeutic Strategies. Semin Oncol. 24: 203–18

Siewert C, Oellinger H, Sherif HK et al. (1997). Is there a Correlation in Breast Carcinomas between Tumor Size and Number of Tumor Vessels detected by Gadolinium-enhanced Magnetic Resonance Mammography? MAGMA 5: 29–31

Stomper PC, Herman S, Klippenstein DL et al. (1996). Invasive Breast Cancer: Analysis of Dynamic Magnetic Resonance Imaging Enhancement Features and Cell proliferative Activity determined by DANN S-phase Percentage. Cancer 77:1844–1849

Stomper PC, Winston JS, Herman S et al. (1997). Angiogenesis and Dynamic MR Imaging Gadolinium Enhancement of Malignant and Benign Breast Lesions. Breast Cancer Res Treat 45:39–46

Weidner N, Semple J, Welch WR, Folkman J (1991). Tumor Angiogenesis and Metastasis-Correlation in Invasive Breast Carcinoma. N Engl J Med 324: 1–8

Weidner N, Folkman J, Pozza F et al. (1992). Tumor Angiogenesis: A new Significant and Independant Prognosic Indicator in Early-Stage Breast Carcinoma. J Natl Cancer Inst 84: 1875–1887

Diagnostic Criteria

Brookes JA, Murray AD, Redpath TW et al. (1996). Choice of Contrast Enhancement Index for Dynamic Magnetic Resonance Mammography. J Magn Reson Imaging 14:1023–1031

Buadu LD, Murakami J, Murayama S et al. (1997). Patterns of Peripheral Enhancement in Breast Masses: Correlation of Findings on Contrast Medium Enhanced MRI with Histologic Features and Tumor Angiogenesis. JCAT 21: 421–430

Buckley DL, Mussurakis S, Horsman A (1998). Effect of Temporal Resolution on the Diagnostic Efficacy of Contrast-Enhanced MRI in the Conservatively Treated Breast. JCAT 22: 47–51

Chenevert TL, Helvie MA, Aisen AM et al. (1995). Dynamic Three-dimensional Imaging with Partial K-Space Sampling: Initial Application for Gadolinium-enhanced Rate Characterization of Breast Lesions. Radiology 196: 135–142

Davis PL, McCarty jr. KS (1997). Sensitivity of Enhanced MRI for the Detection of Breast Cancer: New, Multicentric, Residual, and Recurrent. Eur radiol 7:289–298

Fischer U, von Heyden, Vosshenrich R et al. (1993). Signalverhalten maligner und benigner Läsionen in der dynamischen 2 D-MRT der Mamma. RÖFO 158: 287–292

Friedrich M (1998). MRI of the Breast: State of the Art. Eur Radiol 8:707–725

Gribbestad IS, Nilsen G, Fjosne HE et al. (1994). Comparative Signal Intensity Measurements in Dynamic Gadolinium-enhanced MR-Mammography. JMRI 4: 477–480

Kaiser WA (1993). MR-Mammography (MRM). Springer-Verlag Berlin Heidelberg New York

Kelcz F, Santyr GE, Cron GO, Mongin SJ (1996). Application of a Quantitative Model to Differentiate Benign from Malignant Breast Lesions Detected by Dynamic Gadolinium-enhanced MRI. JMRI 6: 743–752

Kuhl CK, Bieling H, Gieseke J et al. (1997). Breast Neoplasms: $T2^*$ Susceptibility-Contrast, First-Pass Perfusion MR Imaging. Radiology 202: 87–95

Kuhl CK, Klaschik S, Mielcarek P et al. (1999). Do T2-weighted pulse Sequences help with the Differential Diagnosis of Enhancing Lesions in Dynamic Breast MRI? JMRI 9: 187–196

Kuhl CK, Mielcareck P, Klaschik S et al. (1999). Dynamic Breast MR Imaging: Are Signal Intensity Time Course Data Useful for Differential Diagnosis of Enhancing Lesions? Radiology 211: 101–110

Liu PF, Debatin JF, Caduff RF et al. (1998). Improved Diagnostic Accuracy in Dynamic Contrast Enhanced MRI of the Breast by Combined Quantitative and Qualitative Analysis. Brit J Radiol 71:501–509

Mussurakis S, Buckley DL, Drew PJ et al. (1997). Dynamic MR Imaging of the Breast Combined with Analysis of Contrast Agent Kinetics in the Differentiation of Primary Breast Tumor. Clin Radiol 52: 516–526

Mussurakis S, Gibbs P, Horsman A (1998). Peripheral Enhancement and Spatial Contrast Uptake Heterogeneity of Primary Breast Tumours: Quantitative Assessment with Dynamic MRI. JCAT 22: 35–46

Mussurakis S, Gibbs P, Horsman A (1998). Primary Breast Abnormalities: Selective Pixel Sampling on Dynamic Gadolinium-enhanced MR Images. Radiology 206: 465–473

Nunes LW, Schnall MD, Siegelman ES et al. (1997). Diagnostic Performance Characteristics of Architectural Features Revealed by High Spatial-Resolution MR Imaging of the Breast. AJR 169: 409–415

Nunes LW, Schnall MD, Orel SG (1997). Breast MR Imaging: Interpretation Model. Radiology 202: 833–841

Orel SG, Schnall MD, LiVolsi VA, Troupin RH (1994). Suspicious Breast Lesions: MR Imaging with Radiologic-Pathologic Correlation. Radiology 190: 485–493

Piccoli CW (1994). The Specificity of Contrast-enhanced Breast MR Imaging. Magn Reson Imaging Clin N Am 2: 557–571

Piccoli CW (1997). Contrast-enhanced Breast MRI: Factors affecting Sensitivity and Specificity. Eur Radiol 7:281–288

Sherif H, Mahfouz AE, Oellinger H et al. (1997). Peripheral Washout Sign on Contrast-enhanced MR Images of the Breast. Radiology 205: 209–213

Sinha S, Lucas Quesada FA, DeBruhl ND et al. (1997). Multifeature Analysis of Gd-enhanced MR Images of Breast Lesions. JMRI 7: 1016–1026

Stack JP, Redmonds OM, Codd MB et al. (1990). Breast Disease: Tissue Characterization with Gd-DTPA Enhancement Profiles. Radiology 174: 491–494

Weinstein D, Strano S, Cohen P et al. (1999). Breast Fibroadenoma: Mapping of Pathophysiologic Features with Three-Time-Point, Contrast-enhanced MR Imaging-Pilot Study. Radiology 210: 233–240

Sources of Error

Fischer U, Vosshenrich R, Kopka L et al. (1996). Kontrastmittelgestützte dynamische MR Mammographie nach diagnostischen und therapeutischen Eingriffen an der Mamma. Bildgebung 63: 94–100

Heywang-Köbrunner SH (1995). Technique. In: Heywang-Köbrunner SH, Beck R: Contrast-enhanced MRI of the Breast. Springer-Verlag Berlin Heidelberg New York, S. 7–56

Heywang-Köbrunner SH, Wolf HD, Deimling M et al. (1996). Misleading Changes of the Signal Intensity on Opposed-Phase MRI after Injection of Contrast Medium. JCAT 20: 173–178

Kaiser WA (1994). False-positive Results in Dynamic MR-Mammography: Causes, Frequency, and Methods to Avoid. MRI Clin North Amer 2: 539–555

Kaiser WA (1993). Problems and Sources of Error in MRM. In: Kaiser WA: MR-Mammographie (MRM). Springer-Verlag Berlin Heidelberg New York S. 31–35

Peller M, Stehling MK, Sittek H et al. (1996). Effects of Partial Volume and Phase Shift between Fat and Water in Gradient-echo Magnetic Resonance Mammography. MAGMA 4:105–113

Schorn C, Fischer U, Döler W. et al. (1998). Compression Device to Reduce Motion Artifacts at Contrast-enhanced MR Imaging in the Breast. Radiology 206: 279–282

Zuo CS, Jiang A, Buff BL et al. (1996). Automatic Motion Correction for Breast MR Imaging. Radiology 198: 903–906

Normal Findings

Alamo E, Hundertmark C, Fischer U, Grabbe E (1998). KM-gestützte farbkodierte Duplexsonographie bei hypervaskularisierten Herdbefunden in der dynamischen MR-Mammographie. RÖFO 168: S 139

Dean KI, Majurin ML, Komu M. Relaxation Times of Normal Breast Tissue. Acta Radiol 35 (1994) 258–261

Fowler PA, Casey CE, Cameron GG et al. (1990). Cyclic Changes in Composition and Volume of the Breast During the Menstrual Cycle, Measured by Magnetic Resonance Imaging. Br J Obstet Gynecol 97: 595–602

Friedman EP, Hall-Craggs MA, Mumtaz H et al. (1997). Breast MR and the Appearance of the Normal and Abnormal Nipple. Clin Radiol 52: 854–861

Graham SJ, Stanchev PL, Lloyd-Smith JOA et al. (1995). Changes in Fibroglandular Volume and Water Content of Breast Tissue During the Menstrual Cycle Observed by MR Imaging at 1.5 T. JMRI 5: 695–701

Kaiser WA (1987). Die laktierende Mamma im Kernspintomogramm. RÖFO 146: 47–51

Kaiser WA, Mittelmaier O (1992). MR-Mammographie bei Risikopatientinnen. RÖFO 156: 576–581

Kuhl CK, Seibert C, Sommer T et al. (1995). Fokale und diffuse Läsionen in der dynamischen MR-Mammographie gesunder Probandinnen. RÖFO 163: 219–224

Kuhl CK, Bieling H, Gieseke J et al. (1997). Healthy Premenopausal Breast Parenchyma in Dynamic Contrast-enhanced MR Imaging of the Breast: Normal Contrast Medium Enhancement and Cyclical-Phase Dependency. Radiology 203: 137–144

Lee NA, Rusinek H, Weinreb J et al. (1997). Fatty and Fibroglandular Tissue Volumes in the Breasts of Women 20–83 Years Old: Comparison of X-Ray Mammography and Computer-Assisted MR Imaging. AJR 168: 501–506

Martin B, El Yousef SJ (1996). Transverse Relaxation Time Values in MR Imaging of Normal Breast During Menstrual Cycle. JCAT 10: 924–927

Müller-Schimpfle M, Ohmenhäuser K, Claussen CD (1997). Einfluß von Alter und Menstruationszyklus auf Mammographie und MR-Mammographie. Radiologe 37: 718–725

Müller-Schimpfle M, Ohmenhäuser K, Stoll P et al. (1997). Menstrual Cycle and Age: Influence on Parenchymal Contrast Medium Enhancement in MR Imaging of the Breast. Radiology 203: 145–149

Nelson TR, Pretorius DH, Schiffer LM (1985). Menstrual Variation of Normal Breast NMR Relaxation Parameters. JCAT 9: 875–879

Benign Changes

Bässler R (1997). Mamma. In: Remmele W (Hrsg.): Pathologie. Band 4: Weibliches Genitale; Mamma; Pathologie der Schwangerschaft, der Plazenta und des Neugeborenen; Infektionskrankheiten des Fetus und des Neugeborenen; Tumoren des Kindesalters; Endokrine Organe. Springer-Verlag Berlin 133–368

Bassett LW, Jackson VP, Jahan R et al. (1997). Diagnosis of Diseases of the Breast. WB Saunders Philadelphia London Toronto Montreal Sydney Tokyo

Consensus meeting (1986). Is fibrotic Disease of the Breast Precancerous? Arch Pathol Lab Med 110: 171–173

Dupont WD, Page DL (1985) Risk Factors for Breast Cancer in Women with Proliferative Breast Disease. N Engl J Med 312:146

Farria DM, Gorczyca DP, Barsky SH et al. (1996). Benign Phyllodes Tumor of the Breast: MR Imaging Features. AJR 167: 187–189

Fechner RE, Mills SE (1990). Breast Pathology. Benign Proliferations, Atypias and In situ Carcinomas. ASCP Press, Chicago.

Fischer U, Vosshenrich R, von Heyden D et al. (1994). Entzündliche Veränderungen der Mamma – Indikation zur MR-Mammographie? RÖFO 161: 307–311

Fischer U, Kopka L, Brinck U et al. (1997). Prognostic Value of Contrast-enhanced MR-Mammography in Patients with Breast Cancer. Eur Radiol 7: 1002–1005

Friedrich M, Sickles EA (1997). Radiological Diagnosis of Breast Diseases. Springer-Verlag Berlin Heidelberg New York

Harris JR, Lippman ME, Morrow M. Hellman S (1996). Diseases of the Breast. Lippincott-Raven Philadelphia New York

Gallardo X, Sentis M, Castaner E et al. (1998). Enhancement of Intramammary Lymph Nodes with Lymphoid Hyperplasia: A Potential Pitfall in Breast MRI. Eur Radiol 8:1662–1665

Heywang-Köbrunner SH, Beck R (1995). Contrast-enhanced MRI of the Breast. Springer-Verlag Berlin Heidelberg New York

Hochman MG, Orel SG, Powell CM et al. (1997). Fibroadenomas: MR Imaging Appearances with Radiologic-histopathologic Correlation. Radiology 204: 123–129

Kaiser WA (1992). MR-Mammographie bei Risikopatientinnen. RÖFO 156: 576–581

Kaiser WA (1993). MR-Mammography (MRM). Springer-Verlag Berlin Heidelberg New York

Kenzel PP, Hadijuana J, Hosten N et al. (1997). Boeck Sarcoidosis of the Breast. Mammographic, Ultrasound, and MR Findings. JCAT 21: 439–441

Kopans DB (1997). Breast Imaging. Lipincott-Raven Philadelphia New York

Kuhl CK, Bieling H, Gieseke J et al. (1997). Healthy Premenopausal Breast Parenchyma in Dynamic Contrast-enhanced MR Imaging of the Breast: Normal Contrast Medium Enhancement and Cyclicalphase Dependency. Radiology 203: 137–144

Kurtz B, Achten C, Audretsch W et al. (1996). MR-Mammographie der Fettgewebsnekrose. RÖFO 165: 359–363

Ogawa Y, A Nishioka, D Yoshida et al. (1997). Dynamic MR Appearance of Benign Phyllodes Tumor of the Breast in a 20-Year-Old Woman. Radiation Medicine 15: 247–250

Page DL, Dupont WD, Rogers LW, et al. (1985) Atypical Hyperplastic Lesions of the Female Breast: A Long-term Follow-up Study. Cancer 55:2698

Prechtel K (1991). Mastopathie. Histologische Formen und Langzeitbeobachtung. Zbl Pathol 137, 210–215

Rosai J (1996). Ackerman's Surgical Pathology. 8. Auflage. Mosby 1565–1660

Rovno HDS, Siegelman ES, Reynolds C et al. (1998). Solitary Intraductal Papilloma: Findings at MR Imaging and MR Galactography. AJR 1992: 151–155

Sittek K, Kessler M, Heuck AF et al. (1996). Dynamische MR-Mammographie: Ist der Verlauf der Signalintensitätszunahme zur Differenzierung unterschiedlicher Formen der Mastopathie geeignet? RÖFO 165: 59–63

Solomon B, Orel S, Reynolds C, Schnall M (1997). Delayed Development of Enhancement in Fat Necrosis after Breast Conservation Therapy: A Potential Pitfall of MR Imaging of the Breast. AJR 170:966–968

Tomczak R, Rieber A, Zeitler H et al. (1996). Der Wert der MR-Mammographie in der Differentialdiagnostik von nonpuerperaler Mastitis und inflammatorischem Mammakarzinom bei 1,5 T. RÖFO 165: 148–151

Trojani M (1991). A Colour Atlas of Breast Histopathology. 1. Women. Breasts. Diagnosis. Applications of Histopathology. Chapman and Hall Medical London New York Tokyo Melbourne Madras

Unterweger H, Huch Böni RA, Caduff R et al. (1997). Inflammatorisches Mammakarzinom versus puerperale Mastitis. RÖFO 166: 558–560

Weinstein D, Strano S, Cohen P et al. (1999). Breast Fibroadenoma: Mapping of Pathophysiologic Features with Three-Time-Point, Contrast-enhanced MR Imaging-pilot Study. Radiology 210: 233–240

Malignant Changes

Bässler R (1997). Mamma. In: Remmele W (Hrsg.): Pathologie. Band 4: Weibliches Genitale; Mamma; Pathologie der Schwangerschaft, der Plazenta und des Neugeborenen; Infektionskrankheiten des Fetus und des Neugeborenen; Tumoren des Kindesalters; Endokrine Organe. Springer-Verlag Berlin 133–368

Bassett LW, Jackson VP, Jahan R et al. (1997). Diagnosis of Diseases of the Breast. WB Saunders Philadelphia London Toronto Montreal Sydney Tokyo

Boetes C, Mus RDM, Holland R et al. (1995). Breast Tumors: Comparative Accuracy of MR Imaging Relative to Mammography and US for Demonstrating Extent. Radiology 197: 743–747

Boetes C, Strijk SP, Holland R et al. (1997). False-negative MR Imaging of Malignant Breast Tumors. Eur Radiol 7:1231–1234

Boné B, Aspelin P, Bronge L et al. (1996). Sensitivity and Specificity of MR Mammography with Histopathological Correlation in 250 Breasts. Acta Radiol. 37: 208–213

Farria DM, Gorczyca DP, Barsky SH et al. (1996). Benign Phyllodes Tumor of the Breast: MR Imaging Features. AJR 167: 187–189

Fechner RE, Mills SE (1990). Breast Pathology. Benign Proliferations, Atypias and In situ Carcinomas. ASCP Press, Chicago

Fischer U, Westerhof JP, Brinck U et al. (1996). Das duktale In-situ-Karzinom in der dynamischen MR Mammographie bei 1,5 T. RÖFO 164: 290–294

Fischer U, Kopka L, Brinck U et al. (1997). Prognostic Value of contrast-enhanced MR-Mammography in Patients with Breast Cancer. Eur Radiol. 7: 1002–1005

Fischer U, Kopka L, Grabbe E (1996). Invasive Mucinous Carcinoma of the Breast missed by Contrast-enhanced MR Imaging of the Breast. Eur Radiol 6: 929–931

Fischer U, Kopka L, Grabbe E (1999). Therapeutic Impact of Preoperative Contrast-enhanced MR Imaging of the Breast. Radiology (in press)

Friedrich M, Sickles EA (1997). Radiological Diagnosis of Breast Diseases. Springer-Verlag Berlin Heidelberg New York

Gilles R, Guinebretière JM, Lucidarme O et al. (1994). Nonpalpable Breast Tumors: Diagnosis with Contrast-enhanced Subtraction Dynamic MR Imaging. Radiology 191: 625–631

Gilles R, Zafrani B, Guinebretière JM et al. (1995). Ductal carcinoma in Situ: MR Imaging – Histopathologic Correlation. Radiology 196: 415–419

Harms SE, Flamig DP, Hesley KL et al. (1993). MR Imaging of the Breast with Rotating Delivery of Exciting Off Resonance: Clinical Experience with Pathologic Correlation. Radiology 187: 493–501

Harris JR, Lippman ME, Morrow M, Hellman S (1996). Diseases of the Breast. Lippincott-Raven Philadelphia New York

Heinig A, Heywang-Köbrunner SH, Wohlrab J (1997). Seltene Differentialdiagnose einer suspekten Kontrastmittelanreicherung in der Mamma-MRT. Melanommetastase in beiden Mammae. Radiologe 37: 588–590

Hering M, Hagel E, Zwicker C, Krieger G (1996). Bilaterales hochmalignes zentroblastisches Lymphom der Mamma. RÖFO 165: 198–200

Heywang-Köbrunner SH (1993). Brustkrebsdiagnostik mit MR – Überblick nach 1250 Patientenuntersuchungen. Electromedica 61: 43–52

Heywang-Köbrunner SH (1994). Contrast-Enhanced Magnetic Resonance Imaging of the Breast. Invest Radiol 29: 94–104

Heywang-Köbrunner SH, Beck R (1995). Contrast-enhanced MRI of the Breast. Springer-Verlag Berlin Heidelberg New York

Kaiser WA (1993 a). MR-Mammographie. Radiologe 33: 292–299

Kaiser WA (1993 b). MR-Mammographie (MRM). Springer-Verlag Berlin Heidelberg New York

Kenzel PP, Hadijuana J, Hosten N et al. (1997). Boeck Sarcoidosis of the Breast: Mammographic, Ultrasound, and MR Findings. JCAT 21: 439–442

Klengel S, Hietschold V, Schreiber M, Köhler K (1994). Quantitative kontrastmitteldynamische Mamma-MRT am 0,5 Tesla-Gerät. Röntgenpraxis 47: 223–228

Kopans DB (1997). Breast Imaging. Lippincott-Raven Philadelphia New York

Krämer S, Schulz-Wendtland R, Hagedorn K et al. (1998). Magnetic Resonance Imaging and its Role in the Diagnosis of Multicentric Breast Cancer. Anticancer Research 18: 2163–2164

Marchant LK, Orel SG, Perez-Jaffe LA et al. (1997). Bilateral Angiosarcoma of the breast on MR Imaging. AJR 169: 1009–1010

Massurakis S, Carleton PJ, Turnbull LW (1997). MR Imaging of Primary Non-Hodgkin's Breast Lymphoma. Act Radiol 38:104–107

Miller RW, Harms S, Alvarez A (1996). Mucinous Carcinoma of the Breast: Potential False-negative MR Imaging Interpretation. AJR 167: 539–540

Mumtaz H, Hall-Craggs MA, Davidson T et al. (1997). Staging of Symptomatic Primary Breast Cancer with MR Imaging. AJR 169: 417–424

Mussurakis S, Buckley DL, Horsman A (1997). Dynamic MR Imaging of Invasive Breast Cancer: Correlation with Tumour Grade and other Histological Factors. Br J Radiol 70: 446–451

Oellinger H, Heins S, Sander B et al. (1993). Gd-DTPA enhanced MRI of the Breast. The most Sensitive Method for Detecting Multicentric Carcinomas in the Female Breast? Eur Radiol 3: 223–226

Orel SG, Schnall MD, Powell CM et al. (1995). Staging of Suspected Breast Cancer: Effect of MR Imaging and MR-guided Biopsy. Radiology 196: 115–112

Orel SG, Mendonca MH, Reynolds C et al. (1997). MR Imaging of Ductal Carcinoma in Situ. Radiology 202: 413–420

Rieber A, Merkle E, Böhm W et al. (1997). MRI of histologically Confirmed Mammary Carcinoma: Clinical Relevance of Diagnostic Procedures of Detection of Multifocal or Contralateral Secondary Carcinoma. JCAT 21: 773–779

Rieber A, Tomczak RJ, Mergo PJ et al. (1997). MRI of the Breast in the Differential Diagnosis of Mastitis versus Inflammatory Carcinoma and Follow-up. JCAT 21:128–132

Rodenko GN, Harms SE, Pruneda JM et al. (1996). MR Imaging in the Management Before Surgery of Lobular Carcinoma of the Breast: Correlation with Pathology. AJR 167: 1415–1419

Rosai J (1996). Ackerman's Surgical Pathology. 8. Auflage. Mosby 1565–1660

Schorn C, Fischer U, Luftner-Nagel S et al. (1999). MRI of the Breast in Patients with Metastatic Disease of Unknown Primary. Eur Radiol. 9: 470–473

Sittek H, Perlet C, Untch M et al. (1998). Dynamische MR-Mammographie beim invasiv lobulären Mammkarzinom bei 1,0 T. Röntgenpraxis 51: 235–242

Soderstrom CE, Harms SE, Copit DS (1996). Three-dimensional RODEO Breast MR Imaging of Lesions Containing Ductal Carcinoma in Situ. Radiology 201: 427–432

Stomper PC, Herman S, Klippenstein DL et al. (1995). Suspect Breast Lesions: Findings at Dynamic Gadolinium-enhanced MR Imaging Correlated with Mammographic and Pathologic Features. Radiology 197: 387–395

Tessoro-Tess JD, Amoruso A, Rovini D et al. (1995). Microcalcifications in Clinically Normal Breast: The Value of High Field, Surface Coil, Gd-DTPA-enhanced MRI. Eur Radiol 5: 417–422

Teubner J, Back W, Strittmaier HJ et al. (1997). Einseitige Schwellung der Brustdrüse. Radiologe 37: 766–771

Tomczak R, Rieber A, Zeitler H et al. (1996). Der Wert der MR-Mammographie in der Differentialdiagnostik von non-puerperaler Mastitis und inflammatorischem Mammakarzinom bei 1,5 T. RÖFO 165: 148–151

Trojani M (1991). A Colour Atlas of Breast Histopathology. 1. Women. Breasts. Diagnosis. Applications of Histopathology. Chapman and Hall Medical London New York Tokyo Melbourne Madras

Unterweger M, Huch Böni RA, Caduff R et al. (1997). Inflammatorisches Mammakarzinom versus puerperale Mastitis. RÖFO 166: 558–560

Viehweg P, Heinig A, Heywang-Köbrunner et al. (1999). Contrast Enhancement in Dynamic MR Imaging of Noninvasive Breast Cancer. Europ Radiol 9: 260

The Male Breast

Kaiser WA (1993). Breast Diseases in Males. In: WA Kaiser: MR-Mammographie (MRM). Springer-Verlag Berlin Heidelberg New York 1993: 80–81

Indications

Abraham DC, Jones RC, Jones SE et al. (1996). Evaluation of Neoadjuvant Chemotherapeutic Response of Locally advanced Breast Cancer by Magnetic Resonance Imaging. Cancer 78:91–100

Allgayer B, Lukas P, Loos W, Kersting-Sommerhoff B (1993). MRT der Mamma mit 2 D-Spinecho- und Gradientenecho-Sequenzen in diagnostischen Problemfällen. RÖFO 158 423–427

Boetes C, Mus RDM, Holland R et al. (1995). Breast Tumors: Comparative Accuracy of MR Imaging Relative to Mammography and US for Demonstrating Extent. Radiology 197: 743–747

Boné B, Aspelin P, Isberg B et al. (1995). Contrast-Enhanced MR Imaging of the Breast in Patients with Breast Implants after Cancer Surgery. Acta Radiol 36: 111–116

Brenner RJ, Rothman BJ (1997). Detection of Primary Breast Cancer in Women with Known Adenocarcinoma Metastatic to the Axilla Use of MRI after Negative Clinical and Mammographic Examination. J Magn Reson Imaging 7: 1153–1158

Buchberger W, DeKoekkoek-Doll P, Obrist P, Dünser M (1997). Der Stellenwert der MR-Tomographie beim unklaren Mammographiebefund. Radiologe 37: 702–709

Dao TH, Rahmouni A, Campana F et al. (1993). Tumor Recurrence versus Fibrosis in the Irradiated Breast: Differentiation with Dynamic Gadolinium-enhanced MR Imaging. Radiology 187: 751–755

Fischer U, Vosshenrich R, Knipper H et al. (1994): Präoperative MR-Mammographie bei bekanntem Mammakarzinom. Sinnvolle Mehrinformation oder sinnloser Mehraufwand? RÖFO 161: 300–306

Fischer U, Vosshenrich R, von Heyden D et al. (1994). Entzündliche Veränderungen der Mamma – Indikation zur MR-Mammographie? RÖFO 161: 307–311

Fischer U. Vosshenrich R, Kopka L et al. (1996). Kontrastmittelgestützte dynamische MR-Mammographie nach diagnostischen und therapeutischen Eingriffen an der Mamma. Imaging 63: 94–100

Fischer U, Westerhof JP, Brinck U et al. (1996). Das duktale In-situ-Karzinom in der dynamischen MR-Mammographie bei 1,5 T. RÖFO 164: 290–294

Fischer U, Kopka L, Grabbe E (1999). Therapeutic Impact of Preoperative Contrast-enhanced MR Imaging of the Breast. Radiology in press

Gilles R, Guinebretière JM, Shapeero LG et al. (1993). Assessment of Breast Cancer Recurrence with Contrast-enhanced Subtraction MR Imaging: Preliminary Results in 26 Patients. Radiology 188: 473–478

Gilles R, Guinebretière JM, Lucidamre O et al. (1994). Nonpalpable Breast Tumors: Diagnosis with Contrast-enhanced Subtraction Dynamic MR Imaging. Radiology 191: 625–631

Gilles R, Guinebretière JM, Toussaint C et al. (1994). Locally Advanced Breast Cancer: Contrast-enhanced Subtraction MR Imaging of Response to Preoperative Chemotherapy. Radiology 191: 633–638

Harms SE, Flamig DP, Hesley KL et al. (1993) MR Imaging of the Breast with Rotating Delivery of Excitation Off Resonance: Clinical Experience with Pathologic Correlation. Radiology 187: 493–501

Heinig A, Heywang-Köbrunner SH, Viehweg P et al. (1997). Wertigkeit der Kontrastmittel-Magnetresonanztomographie der Mamma bei Wiederaufbau mittels Implantat. Radiologe 37: 710–717

Heywang-Köbrunner SH, Hilbertz T, Beck R et al. (1990). Gd-DTPA Enhanced MR Imaging of the Breast in Patients with Postoperative Scarring and Silicon Implants. JCAT 14: 348–356

Heywang-Köbrunner SH, Beck R (1995). Contrast-enhanced MRI of the Breast. Springer-Verlag Berlin Heidelberg New York

Junkermann H, von Fournier D (1997). Bildgebende Verfahren zur Beurteilung des Ansprechens des Mammakarzinoms auf eine präoperative Chemotherapie. Radiologe 37: 726–732

Kaiser WA (1993). MR-Mammographie (MRM). Springer-Verlag Berlin Heidelberg New York

Knopp MV, Brix G, Junkermann HJ, Sinn HP (1994). MR-Mammographie with Pharmacokinetic Mapping for Monitoring of Breast Cancer Treatment During Neoadjuvant Therapy. MRI Clin North Am 2: 633–658

Krämer S, Schulz-Wendtland R, Hagedorn K et al. (1998 a). Magnetic Resonance Imaging in the Diagnosis of Local Recurrences in Breast Cancer. Anticancer Research 18: 2159–2162

Krämer S, Schulz-Wendtland R, Hagedorn K et al. (1998 b). Magnetic Resonance Imaging and its Role in the Diagnosis of Multicentric Breast Cancer. Anticancer Research 18: 2163–2164

Kuhl CK, Leutner C, Morakkabati N et al. (1999). MR-mammographisches Screening (MRM) bei Hochrisiko-Patientinnen (Trägerinnen des Gens für familiären Brustkrebs, BRCA): Ergebnisse der ersten und zweiten Screening-Runde. RÖFO (in press)

Kurtz B, Achten C, Audretsch W et al. (1996). MR-mammographische Beurteilung des Tumoransprechens nach neoadjuvanter Radiochemotherapie lokal fortgeschrittener Mammakarzinome. RÖFO 164: 469–474

Lagios MD, Westdahl PR, Rose MR (1981). The Concept and Implications of Multicentricity in Breast Carcinoma. Pathol Annu 16: 83–102

Morris EA, Schwartz LH, Dershaw DD et al. (1997). MR Imaging of the Breast in Patients with Occult Primary Breast Carcinoma. Radiology 205: 437–440

Müller RD, Barkhausen J, Sauerwein W, Langer R (1998). Assessment of Local Recurrence after Breast-conserving Therapy with MRI. JCAT 22: 408–412

Mumtaz H, Hall-Craggs MA, Davidson T et al. (1997). Staging of Symptomatic Primary Breast Cancer with MR Imaging. AJR 169: 417–424

Mussurakis H, Davidson T, Hall-Craggs MA et al. (1997). Comparison of Magnetic Resonance Imaging and Conventional Triple Assessment in Locally Recurrent Breast Cancer. Br J Surg 84:1147–1151

Obdejin IMA, Kuipers TJA, van Dijk P et al. (1996). MR Lesion Detection in a Breast Cancer Population. JMRI 6:849–854

Oellinger H, Heins S, Sander B et al. (1993). Gd-DTPA Enhanced MRI of Breast: The Most Sensitive Method for Detecting Multicentric Carcinomas in Female Breast? Eur Radiol 3: 223–226

Orel SG, Schnall MD, Powell CM et al. (1995). Staging of Suspected Breast Cancer: Effect of MR Imaging and MR-Guided Biopsy. Radiology 196: 115–122

Orel SG, Reynolds C, Schnall MD et al. (1997). Breast Carcinoma MR Imaging before Re-excisional Biopsy. Radiology 205: 429–436

Porter BA, Smith JP, Borrwo JW (1995) MR-Depiction of Occult Breast Cancer in Patients with Malignant Axillary Adenopathy. Radiology 1978: 130

Rieber A, Merkle E, Zeitler H et al. (1997). Der unklare Mammabefund – Wert der negativen MR-Mammographie zum Tumorausschluß. RÖFO 167: 392–398

Rieber A, Merkle E, Böhm W et al. (1997). MRI of Histologically Confirmed Mammary Carcinoma: Clinical Relevance of Diagnostic Procedures for Detection of Multifocal or Contralateral Secondary Carcinoma. JCAT 21: 773–779

Rieber A, Merkle E, Zeitler H (1997). Value of MR-Mammography in the Detection and Exclusion of Recurrent Breast Carcinoma. JCAT 21: 780–784

Rieber A, Zeitler H, Rosenthal H et al. (1997). MRI of Breast Cancer: Influence of Chemotherapy on Sensitivity: Br J Radiol 70: 452–458

Rieber A, Zeitler H, Tomczak R et al. (1997). Magnetic Resonance Imaging of the Breast: Changes in Sensitivity during Neoadjuvant Chemotherapy. Br J Radiol 70: 452–458

Rodenko GN, Harms SE, Pruneda JM (1996). MR Imaging in the Management before Surgery of Lobular Carcinoma of the Breast: Correlation with Pathologie. AJR 167: 1415–1419

Schorn C, Fischer U, Luftner-Nagel S et al. (1999). MRI of the Breast in Patients with Metastatic Disease of Unknown Primary. Eur Radiol 9: 470–473

Soderstrom CE, Harms SE, Copit DS (1996). Three-dimensional RODEO Breast MR Imaging of Lesions Containing Ductal Carcinoma in Situ. Radiology 201: 427–432

Soderstrom CE, Harms SE, Farrell RS et al. (1996). Detection with MR Imaging of residual Tumor in the Breast soon after Surgery. AJR 168: 485–488

Tilanus-Linthorst MM, Obdeijn AI, Bontenbal M, Oudkerk M (1997). MRI in Patients with Axillary Metastases of Occult Breast Carcinoma. Breast Cancer Res Treat 44: 179–182

Van Die LE, Boetes C, Barentsz JO, Ruys SH (1996). Additional Value of MR Imaging of the Breast in Women with Pathologic Axillary Lymph Nodes and Normal Mammograms. Radiology 201 (P): 214

Westerhof JP, Fischer U, Moritz JD, Oestmann JW (1998). MR Imaging of Mammographically Detected Clustered Microcalcifications: Is There any Value? Radiology 207: 675–681

Whitehouse GH, Moore NH (1994). MR Imaging of the Breast after Surgery for Breast Cancer. Magn Reson Imaging Clin N Am 2: 591–603

Breast Implants and Plastic Surgery

Ahn CY, Narayanan K, Gorczyca DP et al. (1995). Evaluation of Autogenous Tissue Breast Reconstruction Using MRI. Plast Reconstr Surg 95: 70–76

Azavedo E, Boné B (1999). Imaging Breasts with Silicone Implants. Eur Radiol 9: 349–355

Baker JL, Bartels RJ, Douglas WM (1976). Closed Compression Technique for Rupturing a Contracted Capsule Around a Breast Implant. Plast Reconstr Surg 58: 137–141

Berg WA, Anderson ND, Zerhouni EA et al. (1994). MR Imaging of the Breast in Patients with Silicone Breast Implants: Normal Postoperative Variants and Diagnostic Pitfalls. AJR 163: 575–578

Berg WA, Caskey CI, Hamper UM et al. (1993). Diagnosing Breast Implant Rupture with MR Imaging, US, and Mammography. Radiographics 13: 1323–1336

Berg WA, Caskey CI, Hamper UM et al. (1995). Single- and Double-Lumen Silicone Breast Implant Integrity: Prospective Evaluation of MR and US Criteria. Radiology 197: 45–52

DeAngelis GA, Lange EE, Miller LR, Morgan RF (1994). MR Imaging of Breast Implants. Radiographics 14: 783–794

Everson LI, Parantainen H, Detlie T et al. (1994). Diagnosis of Breast Implant Rupture: Imaging Findings and Relative Efficacies of Imaging Techniques. AJR 163: 57–60

Gorczyca DP, Sinha S, Ahn CY et al. (1992). Silicone Breast Implants in Vivo: MR Imaging. Radiology 185: 407–410

Gorczyca DP (1994). MR Imaging of Breast Implants. MRI Clin North Am 2: 659–672

Gorczyca DP, Brenner RJ (1997). The Augmented Breast. Radiologic & Clinical Perspectives. Thieme New York, Stuttgart

Harms SE, Jensen RA, Meiches MD et al. (1995). Silicone-Suppressed 3 D MRI of the Breast Using Rotating Delivery of Off-Resonance Excitation. JCAT 19: 394–399

Huch RA, Kunzi W, Debatin JF et al. (1998). MR Imaging of the Augmented Breast. Eur Radiol 8:371–376

Kurtz B, Audretsch W, Rezai M et al. (1996). Erste Erfahrungen mit der MR-Mammographie in der Nachsorge bei lappenunterstützter operativer Behandlung des Mammakarzinoms. RÖFO 164: 295–300

Monticciolo DL, Nelson RC, Dixon WT et al. (1994). MR Detection of Leakage from Silicone Breast Implants: Value of a Silicone-selective Pulse Sequence. AJR 163: 51–56

Morgan DE, Kenney PJ, Meeks MC, Pile NS 81996). MR Imaging of Breast Implants and Their Complications. AJR 167: 1271–1275

Mund DF, Farria DM, Gorczyca DP et al. (1993). MR Imaging of the Breast in Patients with Silicone-gel Implants: Spectrum of Findings. AJR 161: 773–778

Piccoli CW, Greer JG, Mitchell DG (1996). Breast MR Imaging for Cancer Detection and Implant Evaluation: Potential Pitfalls. Radiographics 16: 63–75

Soo MS, Kornguth PJ, Walsh R et al. (1996). Complex Radial Folds Versus Subtle Signs of Intracapsular Rupture of Breast Implants: MR Findings with Surgical Correlation. AJR 166: 1421–1427

Stroman PW, Rolland C, Dufour M et al. (1996). Appearance of Low Signal Intensity Lines in MRI of Silicone Breast Implants. Biomaterials 17: 983–988

MR-guided Interventions

Daniel BL, Birdwell RL, Ikeda DM et al. (1998) Breast Lesion Localization: A Freehand, Interactive MR Imaging-guided Technique. Radiology 207: 455–463

Döler W, Fischer U, Metzger I et al. (1996). Stereotaxic Add-on Device for MR-Guided Biopsy of Breast Lesions. Radiology 200: 863–864

Fischer U, Vosshenrich R, Keating D et al. (1994). MR-guided Biopsy of Suspicious Breast Lesions with a Simple Stereotactic Add-on Device for Surface Coils. Radiology 192: 272–273

Fischer U, Vosshenrich R, Bruhn H et al. (1995). MR-Guided Localization of Suspected Breast Lesions Detected Exclusively by Postcontrast MRI. J. Comput Assist Tomo 19: 63–66

Fischer U, Vosshenrich R, Döler W et al. (1995). MR Imaging-guided Breast Intervention: Experience with Two Systems. Radiology 195: 533–538

Fischer U, Rodenwaldt J, Hundertmark C et al. (1997). MRT-gestützte Biopsie und Lokalisation der Mamma. Radiologe 37: 692–701

Gehl HB, Frahm C (1998). MR-gesteuerte Biopsien. Radiologe 38: 194–199

Heinig A, Heywang-Köbrunner SH, Viehweg P et al. (1997). Ein neues Nadelsystem zur MR-gestützten Lokalisation und transkutanen Biopsie von suspekten Befunden in der Brust. In-vitro-Untersuchungen bei 1,0 T.: RÖFO 166: 342–345

Heywang Köbrunner SH, Huynh AT, Viehweg P et al. (1994). Prototype Breast Coil for MR-Guided Needle Localization. JCAT 18: 876–881

Heywang-Köbrunner SH (1996). MR-guided Localization Procedure. In: Heywang-Köbrunner SH, Beck R: Contrast-Enhanced MRI of the Breast. Springer Berlin 1996: 53–56

Heywang-Köbrunner SH, Huynh AT, Viehweg P et al. (1999). MR-guided Percutaneous Vacuum Biopsy of Breast Lesions: Experiences with 60 Cases. Europ Radiol 9 (suppl 1): 195

Kuhl C, Elevelt A, Leutner CC et al. (1997). Interventional Breast MR Imaging: Clinical Use of a Stereotactic Localization and Biopsy Device. Radiology 204: 667–675

Müller-Schimpfle M, Stoll P, Stern W et al. (1998). Präzise MR-gestützte präoperative Markierung von Mammaläsionen mit einer Embolisationsspirale unter Verwendung einer Standard-MR-Spule. RÖFO 168: 195–199

Orel GS, Schnall MD, Newman RW et al. (1994). MR Imaging-guided Localization and Biopsy of Breast Lesions: Initial Experience. Radiology 193: 97–102

Schmitt R, Helmberger T, Fellner F, Obletter N (1993). Markierung nicht-palpabler Mammatumoren in der MRT. Fortschr Röntgenstr. 159: 484–486

Schnall MD, Orel GS, Connick TJ (1994). MR Guided Biopsy of the Breast. In: MRI Clinics of North America. Breast Imaging. 2: 585–589

Sittek H, Kessler M, Müller-Lisse U et al. (1996). Techniken der präoperativen Markierung nicht-palpabler Mammaläsionen in der MRT. RÖFO 165: 84–87

Sittek H, Perlet C, Herrmann K et al. (1997). MR-Mammographie. Präoperative Markierung nichtpalpabler Mammaläsionen am Magnetom Open bei 0,2 T. Radiologe 37: 685–691

DeSouza NM, Coutts GA, Puni RK, Young IR (1996). Magnetic Resonance Imaging Guided Breast Biopsy Using a Frameless Stereotactic Technique. Clin Radiol 51: 425–428

Thiele J, Schneider JP, Franke P et al. (1998). Eine neue Methode der MR-gestützten Mammabiopsie. RÖFO 168: 374–379

Quality Assurance / Perspectives

Daldrup HE, Roberts TPL, Mühler A et al. (1997). Makromolekulare Kontrastmittel für die MR-Mammographie. Ein neuer Ansatz für die Charakterisierung von Mammatumoren. Radiologe 37: 733–740

Daldrup H, Shames DM, Wendland M et al. (1998). Correlation of Dynamic Contrast-enhanced MR Imaging with Histologic Tumor Grade: Comparison of Macromolecular and Small-Molecular Contrast Media. AJR 171: 941–949

Fischer U, Döler W, Luftner-Nagel S et al. (1999). A Multipurpose Phantom for Quality Assurance of Contrast-enhanced MR Imaging of the Breast. Europ Radiol (in press).

Furman-Haran E, Margalit R, Grobgeld D, Degani H (1998). High Resolution MRI of MCF 7 Human Breast Tumors: Complemented Use of Iron Oxide Microsperes and Gd-DTPA. JMRI 8: 634–641

Mumtaz H, Hall-Craggs MA, Wotherspon A et al. (1996). Laser Therapy for Breast Cancer: MR Imaging and Histopathologic Correlation. Adiology 200: 651–658

Westerhof JP, Fischer U, Moritz JD, Oestmann JW (1998). MR Imaging of Mammographically Detected Clustered Microcalcifications: Is there any Value? Radiology 207: 675–681

Index

Note: page numbers in *italics* refer to figures and tables